DIFFERENTIAL DIAGNOSIS FOR THE ADVANCED PRACTICE NURSE

Jacqueline Rhoads, PhD, APRN-BC, CNL-BC, PMHNP-BE, FAANP, is professor of nursing at the University of Texas Medical Branch at Galveston Health Science Center School of Nursing, and has held many faculty positions during her career. Dr. Rhoads has taught in nurse practitioner (NP) programs since 1994. She has been awarded major research funding for a variety of research projects and continues to foster an evidence-based practice implementing outcomes-focused care. Dr. Rhoads earned her PhD from the University of Texas, Austin, and has earned postmaster's degrees in acute care, community health primary care, adult nursing practice, gerontology, and psychiatric/mental health nursing practices and, recently, her clinical nurse leader certification. She is a fellow in the American Academy of Nurse Practitioners, and was awarded numerous commendations and medals for meritorious service in the U.S. Army Nurse Corps. Dr. Rhoads has authored three books for major nursing publishers as well as numerous articles. Her most recent publication *Nurses' Clinical Consult to Psychopharmacology* (2012) won first place as AJN Book of the Year Award. Her textbook *Clinical Consult to Psychiatric Mental Health Care* won second place as AJN Book of the Year Award in 2011.

Marilee Murphy Jensen, MN, ARNP, is a family NP (FNP) with more than 20 years of clinical experience as well as more than 16 years of experience as a lecturer and clinician teacher. Ms. Jensen currently is director of the Family Nurse Practitioner Program at Seattle University College of Nursing, where she coordinates the program and teaches in all aspects of family practice. Her clinical affiliation is with the Medical Arts Clinic, Family Practice in Bellevue, Washington. Previous faculty appointments include positions at the University of Washington School of Nursing (Seattle) and the University of Victoria (British Columbia, Canada). Prior to becoming an FNP in 1988, Marilee had 15 years of RN experience in medical, surgical, critical care intensive care unit, and emergency room areas. Her FNP experience includes in-depth clinical work in gynecology, urgent care, internal medicine, rheumatology, asthma, and family practice. Honors include Preceptor of the Year (University of Washington, School of Nursing in 2003) and nominations for Distinguished Faculty of the Year (University of Washington, School of Nursing, 2001, 2002, and 2003). She is certified as an FNP by the American Nurses Credentialing Center (ANCC) and is licensed as an FNP in both Washington State and Oregon.

DIFFERENTIAL DIAGNOSIS FOR THE ADVANCED PRACTICE NURSE

Jacqueline Rhoads, PhD, APRN-BC, CNL-BC, PMHNP-BE, FAANP

Marilee Murphy Jensen, MN, ARNP

Editors

SPRINGER PUBLISHING COMPANY

NEW YORK

Springer Publishing Company, LLC
11 West 42nd Street
New York, NY 10036
www.springerpub.com

Acquisitions Editor: Margaret Zuccarini
Composition: Exeter Premedia Services Private Ltd.

ISBN: 978-0-8261-1027-5
e-book ISBN: 978-0-8261-1028-2

15 16 17 / 5 4 3 2

The author and the publisher of this Work have made every effort to use sources believed to be reliable to provide information that is accurate and compatible with the standards generally accepted at the time of publication. The author and publisher shall not be liable for any special, consequential, or exemplary damages resulting, in whole or in part, from the readers' use of, or reliance on, the information contained in this book. The publisher has no responsibility for the persistence or accuracy of URLs for external or third-party Internet websites referred to in this publication and does not guarantee that any content on such websites is, or will remain, accurate or appropriate.

Library of Congress Cataloging-in-Publication Data
Differential diagnosis for the advanced practice nurse / Jacqueline Rhoads, Marilee Murphy Jensen, editors.
    p. ; cm.
  ISBN 978-0-8261-1027-5—ISBN 978-0-8261-1028-2 (e-book)
  I. Rhoads, Jacqueline, 1948– editor.   II. Jensen, Marilee Murphy, editor.
  [DNLM: 1. Nursing Diagnosis—methods.   2. Diagnosis, Differential.   3. Physical Examination—nursing.
  WY 100.4]
  RT48
  616.07'5—dc23
                                                                    2014012240

Special discounts on bulk quantities of our books are available to corporations, professional associations, pharmaceutical companies, health care organizations, and other qualifying groups. If you are interested in a custom book, including chapters from more than one of our titles, we can provide that service as well.

For details, please contact:
Special Sales Department, Springer Publishing Company, LLC
11 West 42nd Street, 15th Floor, New York, NY 10036-8002
Phone: 877-687-7476 or 212-431-4370; Fax: 212-941-7842
E-mail: sales@springerpub.com

vii, 236
Printed in the United States of America by Gasch Printing.

6/3/15

CONTENTS

CONTRIBUTORS

Patricia Abbott, PhD, MSN, FNP-C   Assistant Professor, Regis University College of Nursing, Lakewood, Colorado

Barbara Bjeletich, ARNP   Emergency Room Provider, University of Washington, Seattle, Washington

Dorothy Cooper, MN, ARNP, ANP-BC, WHNP-BC   Nurse Practitioner, The Everett Clinic, Everett, Washington

Patricia Cox, DNP, MPH, FNP-BC   Assistant Professor, DNP Clinical Coordinator, University of Portland, School of Nursing, Portland, Oregon

John Cranmer, DNP, MPH, MSN, ANP-BC   Senior Research Fellow, Department of Global Health, University of Washington, Internal Medicine Nurse Practitioner, SeaMar Community Health Centers, Seattle, Washington

Lynda Hillman, DNP, FNP-BC   Nurse Practitioner, Multiple Sclerosis Center/ Rehabilitation Medicine, University of Washington Medical Center, Seattle, Washington

Marilee Murphy Jensen, ARNP, MSN   Family Nurse Practitioner, Northwest Hospital, University of Washington, Seattle, Washington

Sarah Kooienga, PhD, ARNP, FNP   Assistant Professor, Washington State University College of Nursing, Vancouver, Washington

Patricia Mathis, MSN, FNP-BC   Issaquah, WA

Melody Rasmor, EdD(c), APRN-BC, COHN-S   Assistant Professor, Washington State University College of Nursing, Vancouver, Washington

Jacqueline Rhoads, PhD, APRN-BC, CNL-BC, PMHNP- BE, FAANP   Professor, Graduate Nursing Department, University of Texas Medical Branch School of Nursing, Galveston, Texas

Christie Rivelli, MSN, FNP   Family Nurse Practitioner, Coastal Family Health Center, Battle Ground, Washington

Kumhee Ro, DNP, ARNP, FNP   Clinical Assistant Professor, Biobehavioral Nursing and Health Systems, School of Nursing, University of Washington, Seattle, Washington

Melody Stringer, MSN, ARNP-BC   Nurse Practitioner, The Vancouver Clinic (Urgent Care), Vancouver, Washington

Diane Switzer, DNP, ARNP, FNP-BC, ENP-BC, CCRN, CEN   Emergency Department, Harborview Medical Center, University of Washington, Bellevue, Washington

Charles Wiley, MSN, ARNP, FNP-BC   Adjunct Faculty, Puget Sound Physicians Group, Emergency Department, Harborview Medical Center, University of Washington, Bellevue, Washington, Adjunct Faculty, Seattle Pacific University ARNP Program, Issaquah, Washington

PREFACE

Establishing *differential diagnosis* can be challenging even for the expert advanced practice nurse (APN). For the APN student, establishing the diagnosis is even more of a challenge. It is the goal of the authors to present a clinically useful guide for both the student and the clinical provider to use in discerning a reliable diagnosis. Much of the diagnosis is based on patient input, so standard methods of communicating with the patient are important in eliciting a useful history and background that can accurately point the APN to a likely diagnosis. Using this as a platform from which to conduct and order appropriate diagnostic tests is the next logical step for the clinician. How does one learn to formulate such a platform? Currently, there are very few textbooks available that would provide such a guide to the development of a differential diagnosis for common patient/client complaints. This book is designed to bridge the gap between common chief complaints and the formulation of a correct diagnosis by providing a step-by-step approach to eliciting useful patient responses through an unfolding case study approach. We have attempted to include the more commonly occurring symptoms that present in the clinical setting. There are a few symptoms such as "fever" that have been omitted, as this "symptom" might require an entire treatise on its own if we were to address every possible condition that included fever as part of the presenting symptoms.

This handy clinical reference presents a standard method of formulating a differential diagnosis that the APN can use throughout clinical practice. Thirty-eight common symptoms are organized and presented in alphabetical order, starting with abdominal pain and moving through to cough, ear discharge, fatigue, hand and joint swelling, headache, low back pain, shortness of breath, and skin rashes, to vomiting and wrist pain (last symptom). These symptoms, or chief complaints, represent the symptoms most frequently presented by patients to the primary care practitioner.

PATIENT-BASED CASE SCENARIOS

The patient-based case scenario is used to present each symptom. The case unfolds systematically and is followed consistently as each symptom is explored, as in a clinical setting. This systematic approach helps the student to structure her or his approach to a patient, supporting the idea of establishing a method of clinical decision making. Each symptom exploration follows the same format, which includes a "Case Presentation" followed by:

1. Introduction to Complaint (includes background, usual cause, additional causes)
2. History of Complaint (includes symptomatology, directed questions to ask, assessment: cardinal signs and symptoms, medical history: general, medical history: specific to complaint)

3. Physical Examination (includes vital signs, general appearance, visual examination of area concerning chief complaint, additional related inspection and examination, areas to palpate and areas to auscultate)
4. Case Study: History and Physical Examination Findings (includes responses to directed questions, findings of physical examination)
5. Differential Diagnosis (a table that compares typical symptoms associated with conditions that might present similarly and need to be compared with the results of the patient's history and physical examination findings)
6. Diagnostic Examination (a table that presents diagnostic tests that the APN can consider performing or ordering to facilitate arriving at the correct diagnosis)
7. Clinical Decision Making (a summary of the case study and statement of the likely diagnosis)

UNIQUE FEATURES

Case Study: History—This two-column table presents the directed question posed to the patient in the first column and the patient's response to the question in the second column.

Case Study: Physical Examination Findings—This section presents the actual findings of the physical examination. Together, the case study history table and the case study physical examination findings lead the examiner to the differential diagnosis table, which clearly compares the relative differences among the more usual and customary diagnoses.

Differential Diagnosis Table—This table presents the more usual diagnostic choices that can be made based on the client's chief complaint and provides the clinician significant clues as to which diagnoses might be most accurate.

Diagnostic Examination Table—This table presents the diagnostic tools available to further clarify or confirm a diagnosis related to the presenting symptom. It includes the estimated cost and codes to be considered when determining which tests to order. Some of the tests are common tests that are included in the office visit, such as the otoscopy, which provides visualization of the ear canal and tympanic membrane to assess for the presence of foreign body, signs of trauma, erythema, effusion, or rupture. Others provide more insight into a possible diagnosis and often are more costly.

Clinical Decision Making—This section describes the APN's analysis of the patient's health history (including responses to directed and nondirected questions), the physical exam, results of the diagnostic tests, and the scrutiny of the differential diagnosis table (comparing common symptoms for possible diagnoses). Decision making is laid out for the reader, indicating the salient points that surfaced during the analysis process, and offers the most likely diagnosis.

Clinical information presented in this book is considered generally accepted practice. Although every effort has been made to present correct and up-to-date information, the health care field is rapidly changing and the idea of "common knowledge" today might be different tomorrow, based on new developments and research findings. For this reason, readers are encouraged to keep up with all available resources to help ensure accurate decision making.

Establishing differential diagnoses for client complaints is a critical step in the delivery of optimum health care. It is our hope that this book will serve as a useful guide for nurses in practice. We feel it will be a wonderful adjunct to APN curricula in nursing programs across the globe.

Jacqueline Rhoads
Marilee Murphy Jensen

ACKNOWLEDGMENTS

I would like to express my gratitude to the many people who saw me through this book; to all those who provided support, talked things over, read, wrote, offered comments, allowed me to quote their remarks, and assisted in the editing, proofreading, and design.

I would like to thank Chris Teja for helping me in the process of topic selection and editing. Thanks to Margaret Zuccarini, my editor, who encouraged me. Without them this book would have never found its way to the advanced practice faculty and providers.

Above all, I want to thank my mother, who supported and encouraged me in spite of all the time it took me away from her.

Jacqueline Rhoads

INTRODUCTION TO DIFFERENTIAL DIAGNOSIS AND DIAGNOSIS OF COMMON PROBLEMS

Diseases are defined by a pattern of symptoms the patient reports, signs observed during physical examination, and diagnostic testing. Determining the differential diagnosis is the process of distinguishing one disease from another that presents with similar symptoms. With the chief complaint established, information is gathered through the history and physical examination. When the patient presents with a chief complaint, such as cough, the provider considers the most common diseases that present with cough, forming a working differential diagnosis list. The provider analyzes the data obtained, eliminates some diseases, and narrows down the differential diagnosis. At times, further diagnostic testing is needed to make the final diagnosis. The construction of a differential diagnosis is essential in making an accurate diagnosis.

PATIENT HISTORY
Identification/Chief Complaint

The first piece of information obtained is the chief complaint or the patient's reason for seeking medical attention. This statement gives the provider a general idea of possible diagnoses. For example, "a healthy 16-year-old boy presents with a nonproductive cough for 3 days."

Subjective

The most common etiology of the disease is in the ears, nose, throat, and respiratory system. With this in mind, the provider asks the patients a series of *open-ended questions* to gather data related to the presenting problem. These questions form the basis of the symptom analysis:

- Onset
- Location/radiation
- Duration/timing
- Character
- Associated symptoms
- Aggravating or triggering factors
- Alleviating factors
- Effects on daily life

Once a general history is obtained, the provider moves on to obtain more details through a *directed history*. Patients may not offer pertinent symptoms unless prompted. These questions are focused on the diagnostic possibilities related to the presenting problem. For example, a patient who presents with chest pain may not recall that the pain is much better when he or she leans forward, indicating possible pericarditis.

Once questions regarding the symptom are completed, the provider moves on to obtain data regarding the patient's general health status, and relevant past medical, family, and social history. The patient's past medical history and family history outline risk factors for diseases. The social history may reveal occupational exposures or habits that influence the presence of diseases, such as heart and lung disease from smoking, or liver disease from alcohol or drug use.

PHYSICAL EXAMINATION

The physical examination starts when you walk into the room and observe the patient's general appearance. Visual clues include facial expression, mood, stress level, hygiene, skin color, and breathing pattern. Although they may seem trivial, the assessment of vital signs is critical, and their accuracy is imperative. The presence of fever, tachycardia, or low blood pressure is cause for concern and alerts the provider that the patient may have a serious disease.

Unlike the patient who comes in for a comprehensive physical examination, the patient who presents with a symptom requires a *focused* physical examination. The examination is directed by the chief complaint and history. For example, a 16-year-old with a recent cough requires examination of the ears, eyes, nose, throat, neck (for lymphadenopathy), heart, lungs, and abdomen (for an enlarged liver or spleen). Attention is given to the skin to look for cyanosis, the nails for clubbing, and the vascular system for edema. Neurologic examination is limited to mental status, and other parts of the examination are not relevant.

The physical examination provides positive and negative findings, and may provide the diagnosis without the need for further testing. For example, if the examination of a patient who reports a painful skin rash yields findings of a cluster of vesicles on an erythematous base following a dermatome, this is a positive physical finding confirming clinical diagnosis of herpes zoster. On the other hand, the lack of a rash would be a negative physical finding and further exploration is needed. The physical examination may also reveal unsuspected findings, or may be completely normal despite the presence of disease.

DIFFERENTIAL DIAGNOSIS

Once the chief complaint, history, and physical examination are established, a list of possible diseases is formed ranking the most common diagnoses and the most serious or "not to miss" diagnoses. The axiom that common diseases present commonly and uncommon diseases are uncommon cannot be overstressed. Keeping an open mind, and exploring all possibilities, is important. Premature closure or discarding a diagnosis too early may result in diagnostic error. The depth of one's differential diagnosis is determined by the breadth of knowledge of the provider. A disease cannot be diagnosed and treated unless it is known to the provider. This can be a challenge for the novice who is faced with a mountain of information to learn about thousands of diseases. It results in a chronic sense of dissatisfaction with one's knowledge base, and can be a source of great fear and frustration. However, it serves to stimulate exploration and learning, and with experience and guidance, knowledge grows. The novice will find that a solid reference enables him or her to master the task of differential diagnosis as his or her clinical experience matures.

DIAGNOSTIC TESTING

When the diagnosis cannot be made on history and physical data alone, diagnostic testing is the next step in determining the correct diagnosis. Diagnostic testing should be done only if necessary to yield an impact on the diagnosis, and ultimate treatment of the problem. Ordering unnecessary tests is enormously expensive. When possible, order basic tests to screen for disease, and if the diagnosis remains unclear, move on to more elaborate testing.

Consider the sensitivity and specificity of a test as well. "Sensitivity" is the proportion of patients with the diagnosis who will test positive. "Specificity" is the proportion of patients without the diagnosis who will test negative.

If the diagnosis is not defined by the history, physical examination, and diagnostic testing, the provider then needs to reevaluate the patient over time, reformulating new diagnostic possibilities as new signs or symptoms arise.

STEPS TO WRITING A DIFFERENTIAL DIAGNOSIS

Knowledge of how to write a medical diagnosis comprises several critical steps.

1. Obtain the patient's chief complaint, such as "cough for 2 weeks" and list three common problems that present with that symptom. For example, acute cough is most likely viral bronchitis, pneumonia, or viral rhinosinusitis with postnasal drip.
2. Obtain a detailed history as outlined above. Make a list of the patient's symptoms and pertinent risk factors. Note the pertinent positive and negative associated symptoms. For example, a patient with a cough who has a high fever and shortness of breath (positives) likely has pneumonia. A patient who has a cough without a high fever or shortness of breath (negatives) may have a viral bronchitis. Based on the information from your history, direct your physical examination to look for significant signs of illness. For example, is there sinus tenderness? Is there a postnasal drip in the posterior pharynx? Are there wheezes or crackles present?
3. Review your differential diagnosis list of possible diagnoses based on the history and physical examination. Determine whether you need additional diagnostic testing based on your findings. For example, a patient with a fever of 102°F, heart rate of 120, and respiratory rate of 30 with diminished breath sounds in the right lower lobe and crackles will benefit from a chest x-ray to confirm the presence or absence of pneumonia. A complete blood count will identify whether there is a significant leukocytosis or elevated white blood cell count. A basic metabolic panel will ascertain whether there is an electrolyte imbalance or dehydration.
4. Establish a clear determination that shows why this particular diagnosis is accurate for the patient. Review your rationale for why you chose this diagnosis as opposed to others on your list of possibilities. Keep an open mind as you review your facts for any other diagnostic possibilities you may have missed, including a life-threatening illness.
5. Develop a treatment plan, including diagnostic testing, pharmacologic agents, patient education, and follow-up. If your diagnosis remains unclear, consider appropriate referral for further evaluation.

SUMMARY

This book is written to help the reader learn the process of formulating a differential diagnosis using the skills of gathering appropriate data from the history, physical examination, and relevant diagnostic testing. Each chapter is interspersed with cases describing an initial chief complaint, history, and physical examination. Tables outlining the common diagnosis with cardinal signs and symptoms as well as diagnostic testing are provided for the reader's review. Clinical diagnostic reasoning for the final diagnosis is outlined. The approach is to give pertinent information as well as demonstrate the process of clinical reasoning. It is well known that the process of differential diagnosis takes years to master. It is especially challenging for new students learning the complexities of diagnosis. It is my hope that this book will help you start your journey with the tools to make this learning process interesting and relevant.

ABDOMINAL PAIN

Case Presentation: A 25-year-old female presents to the emergency room (ER) with complaints of severe abdominal pain.

INTRODUCTION TO COMPLAINT

- Abdominal pain is a subjective feeling of discomfort in the abdomen
- It is caused by a variety of problems
- The goal of the initial assessment is to distinguish acute life-threatening conditions from chronic/recurrent or mild, self-limiting conditions
- It can be caused by tension in the gastrointestinal (GI) tract
  - Muscle contraction or distention
  - Ischemia
  - Inflammation of the peritoneum

Colic Pain

- Tension-type pain
- Associated with forceful peristaltic contractions
- Most characteristic type of pain arising from the viscera
- Produced by an irritant substance, from infection or bacteria, or the body's attempt to force its luminal contents through an obstruction

Stretching Pain

- Tension-type pain
- Caused by acute stretching of an organ, such as the liver, spleen, or kidney, due to enlargement
- Patient is restless, moves about, and has difficulty getting comfortable

Ischemic Pain

- Intense, continuous pain
- Strangulation of bowel from obstruction is a common cause

Inflammatory Pain

- Visceral peritonitis
- Aching
- Patient lies still and does not want to move
- Pain may be referred from abdomen to other parts of the body via common neural pathways

HISTORY OF COMPLAINT
Symptomatology

Ask about the following characteristics of each symptom using open-ended questions:

- Onset (sudden or gradual)
- Chronology
- Current situation (improving or deteriorating)
- Location
- Radiation
- Quality
- Timing (frequency, duration)
- Severity
- Precipitating and aggravating factors
- Relieving factors
- Associated symptoms
- Effects on daily activities
- Previous diagnosis of similar episodes
- Previous treatments
- Efficacy of previous treatments

Directed Questions to Ask

- How long ago did your pain start?
- Was the onset gradual or sudden?
- What word would describe your pain; is it dull, sharp, crampy, or grabbing?
- Does your pain come and go or is it constant?
- How long does it last?
- Is the pain getting worse?
- Does your pain radiate into your back, groin, or legs?
- Do you have a change in your appetite?
- Do you have any nausea, or vomiting?
- Do you have any burning in the abdomen or chest?
- Do you have any constipation or diarrhea?
- Do you have any pain or difficulty with urination?
- Have you had any blood in your urine?
- Have you been sexually active?
- Have you had any pain with sexual activity?
- When was your last menstrual period?
- Have you missed any periods?
- Have you had any abnormal spotting?
- Have you had any vaginal discharge that is different from your usual?
- Is there any vaginal odor?
- Have you had any new stressors or life changes prior to your new onset of pain?

Assessment: Cardinal Signs and Symptoms

In addition to the general characteristics outlined above, the location of the pain provides an important clue to the possible etiology of the pain.

Pain Location
- EPIGASTRIC: esophagus, stomach, duodenum, liver, gallbladder, pancreas, spleen
- UPPER ABDOMINAL: esophagus, stomach, duodenum, liver, gallbladder, pancreas, thorax

- RIGHT UPPER QUADRANT (RUQ): usually esophagus, stomach, duodenum, liver, gallbladder, pancreas, thorax; often indicates cholecystitis
- LEFT UPPER QUADRANT (LUQ): spleen

Medical History: General

- Medical conditions and surgeries
- Allergies
- Current medications
- Bowel pattern
- Last menstrual period (LMP)

Medical History: Specific to Complaint

- Previous abdominal surgeries
- Pregnancies
- Miscarriages
- Abortions
- Recent use of new prescribed medications
- Recent use of over-the-counter medications, such as ibuprofen or naprosyn
- Family history of cancer of the stomach, bowel, uterus, or ovaries

PHYSICAL EXAMINATION

Vital Signs

- Temperature
- Pulse
- Respiration
- Oxygen saturation (SpO_2)
- Blood pressure (BP)

General Appearance

- Apparent state of health
- Appearance of comfort or distress
- Color
- Nutritional status
- Hygiene
- Match between appearance and stated age
- Difficulty with gait or balance

Abdominal Inspection
- SKIN: color, lesions, masses, or hernias
- SIZE/SHAPE: distention, shape, symmetry, surgical scars, hernias, pulsations

Abdominal Examination
- AUSCULTATION: for frequency, intensity, pitch of bowel sounds, determine presence of bruits, friction rub
- RECTAL: if rectal bleeding or change in bowel habits; testing of hemocult as positive or negative

Pelvic Examination
- EXTERNAL: observe for redness or lesions
- INTROITUS: observe for discharge or lesions
- VAGINA: observe for presence or absence of rugae, discharge, bleeding, or odor

- CERVIX: inspect for lesions, discharge from os; note whether there is pain with motion of the cervix from side to side
- UTERUS: note size, shape, and position and whether there is any tenderness with movement
- OVARIES: note if palpable; if palpable, note whether they are enlarged, tender, or masses are present
- PERCUSSION: look for patterns of dullness and tympany
- PALPATION: locate masses or organomegaly, pulsations
  - Light palpation: tenderness, pain, presence of guarding, rigidity, and rebound tenderness
  - Deep palpation: locate masses or organomegaly, pulsations

CASE STUDY
History

Question	Response
When did the pain start?	*2 weeks ago*
On a scale of 0 to 10 what number would you give the intensity of the pain?	*8 to 10*
Is the pain sharp, dull, or crampy?	*The pain is sharp and crampy*
Is it constant or does it come and go?	*It comes and goes?*
What triggers the pain?	*It hurts if I run, sit down hard, or if I have sex*
Do you have any nausea or vomiting?	*No*
How is your appetite?	*It is good*
Do you have constipation or diarrhea?	*No*
Do you have fever or chills?	*No*
When was your last period?	*5 days ago*
Was it at the normal time?	*Yes*
Are you using birth control?	*Yes, I take the shot each month*
Was your period associated with more pain or cramping?	*Yes, it was the worst period pain I ever had*
Have you ever had an infection in your ovary or uterus before?	*No, never*
Have you ever been pregnant?	*No, never*
Have you had a new partner?	*Yes, we started up about 2 months ago*
Do you feel safe with your new partner?	*Yes, he's really good to me*
Do you use condoms?	*No, he hates them*
Do you have anything else to tell me?	*No, I just want to get rid of this pain*

Physical Examination Findings

- VITAL SIGNS: BP 138/90; temperature 99°F; respiratory rate (RR) 20; heart rate (HR) 110, regular; oxygen saturation (PO_2) 96%; pain 5/10
- GENERAL APPEARANCE: female in acute distress and severe pain
- HEAD, EYES, EARS, NOSE, THROAT (HEENT): within normal limits; eyes: anicteric; pupils equal, round, and reactive to light and accommodation (PERRLA); nose: no discharge; mouth/throat: moist membranes, no lesions
- CHEST: lung clear in all fields; S1S2, no murmurs, gallops, or rubs
- ABDOMEN: soft, diffuse tenderness
- SKIN: no rashes
- EXTREMITIES: range of motion (ROM) × 4, no joint pain or swelling

Abdominal Examination

- INSPECTION: no masses or thrills noted; no discoloration and skin is warm to; no tattoos or piercings; abdomen is nondistended and round
- AUSCULTATION: bowel sounds (BS) are normal in all four quadrants, no bruits noted
- PALPATION: on palpation, abdomen is tender to touch in four quadrants; tenderness noted on light palpation, deep palpation reveals no masses, spleen and liver unremarkable
- PERCUSSION: tympany heard in all quadrants, no dullness noted in abdominal area

Pelvic Examination

- EXTERNAL: mature hair distribution; no external lesions on labia
- INTROITUS: slight green-gray discharge, no lesions
- VAGINAL: normal rugae; moderate amount of green discharge on vaginal walls
- CERVIX: nulliparous os with small amount of purulent discharge from os with positive cervical motion tenderness (CMT)
- UTERUS: ante-flexed, normal size, shape, and position
- ADNEXA: bilateral tenderness with fullness; both ovaries without masses
- RECTAL: deferred
- VAGINAL DISCHARGE: green in color

DIFFERENTIAL DIAGNOSIS

Differential Diagnosis	Pelvic Inflammatory Disease	Sexually Transmitted Disease	Septic Abortion	Ectopic Pregnancy	Appendicitis
Onset	Gradual	Gradual	Sudden	Sudden	Sudden
Pain	+	+	+	+	+
Location	Pelvic area/ right and left lower quadrant	Pelvic area/ right and left lower quadrant	Localized	Pelvic area/ right and left lower quadrant	Epigastric or per umbilical/ right lower quadrant
Fever	High	High or low	High	If ruptured	Possible
Discharge	Common	Common	Common with infection	Possible	–

(continued)

Differential Diagnosis	Pelvic Inflammatory Disease	Sexually Transmitted Disease	Septic Abortion	Ectopic Pregnancy	Appendicitis
Inguinal nodes	+	+	+	+	+
Vaginal bleeding	Possible	Rare	Common	Common	–
CMT	Very common	Common	Common	Common	–

DIAGNOSTIC EXAMINATION

Examination	Procedure Code	Cost	Results
Complete blood count (CBC) with differential	85025	$75	High white blood cells (WBCs)
Quantitative pregnancy test	81025		Done to rule out the possibility of a tubal/ectopic pregnancy
Wet mount (saline)	87070	$23.26	If pH < 4.5, wet mount reveals up to 3 to 5 WBCs/high power field and presence of epithelial cells and lactobacilli (may be physiological discharge) WBCs high in the presence of a foreign body
Chlamydia and gonococcus (sexually transmitted disease [STD] test)	V73.88, V74.5	$28 each	Common link to PID
Urinalysis and urine culture if urinalysis (UA) shows leukocytes	81000	$55	Screens for infection
Pelvic and vaginal ultrasound	76830	$390	Examines margins of pelvic structures to determine size
Culdocentesis	57020	$125	Determines hemoperitoneum (ruptured ectopic pregnancy from pelvic sepsis)
Laparoscopy	58541–58544	$1700	Definitive test to diagnose PID but due to invasiveness it is not done often Usually indicated when the diagnosis is in doubt or the results of the procedure are questionable

CLINICAL DECISION MAKING
Case Study Analysis

Pertinent positives are:

- Fever, lower abdominal pain above pubic bone that is band-like
- Dyspareunia
- Greenish vaginal discharge with dysuria
- Burning on urination

Pertinent negatives are:

- Normal, regular menses
- Negative pregnancy test
- No fever or chills

> ***Diagnosis:*** *Pelvic inflammatory disease*

FURTHER READING

Barad, D. H. (2012). *Vaginal itching and discharge.* Retrieved from http://www.merckmanuals.com /professional/gynecology_and_obstetrics/symptoms_of_gynecologic_disorders/vaginal_itching _and_discharge.html

National Guideline Clearinghouse. (2010). Diseases characterized by vaginal discharge. In *Sexually transmitted diseases treatment guidelines.* Retrieved from http://www.guidelines.gov/content .aspx?id=2558

Rhoads, J., & Petersen, S. (2013). *Advanced health assessment and diagnostic reasoning.* Sudbury, MA: Jones & Bartlett.

ANKLE PAIN

Case Presentation: *A 48-year-old avid female runner presents to your clinic with a complaint of ankle pain on the left ankle for 3 days.*

INTRODUCTION TO COMPLAINT

- The ankle is a base, a lever, and a shock absorber
- Ankle pain can be acute or chronic
- Acute pain is usually caused by an injury due to ankle ligament injuries
- Assessment of acute ankle pain should be focused on the mechanism of injury
- The necessity for radiography is determined by clinical presentation
- When pain and swelling have diminished, reexamination 3 to 5 days later is completed for differentiating diagnosis of a partial tear from frank ligament rupture. Assessment before that time could be inconclusive.

Acute Pain

- Fracture
- Trauma to the ligament or tendon
- Inflammation due to arthritis or bursitis

Chronic Pain

- Most often caused by degenerative joint disease, usually osteoarthritis
- Is a slow progression, not a result of recent injury or trauma
- Overuse of the joint can cause inflammation and edema and some inflammation to the bursa can be involved
- Could be infectious (osteonecrosis)
- Could be related to loss of bone due to metabolic disorders as with parathyroid disease, osteoporosis, and Paget's disease

HISTORY OF THE COMPLAINT
Symptomatology

Ask about the following characteristics of each symptom using open-ended questions:

- Determine the onset and mechanism of the injury
- The mechanism of injury is helpful in guiding decision making
- The ankle is a complex joint; the two directions of injury include
  - Inversion/supination and eversion/pronation
    - Stretched areas usually fracture or tear prior to those being compressed
    - With an inversion injury the lateral ankle is stretched
    - In an eversion injury the medial aspect is stretched

- Internal and external rotation of the talus: The rotational forces stress supporting structures and can guide injury examination
- The position of the ankle at the time of the injury
- The force applied to the ankle that causes the injury
- The amount of force

Directed Questions to Ask

- How did you injure your ankle?
- Where is the site of the most significant pain?
- Do you have other injured areas on the body (hip, knee)?
- How long has it been since the injury?
- Can you put weight on it? Range of motion; none to full?
- Neurovascular symptoms: Any numbness or tingling or other symptoms characteristic of compartment syndrome?
- History of injury or intervention to lower extremities?
- Related conditions:
  - Do you smoke?
  - High body mass?
  - Do you have diabetes?
  - Are you on chronic steroids?
- What medications have you taken for systemic disease or previous ankle injury or disability?

Assessment: Cardinal Signs and Symptoms

- Does the patient need surgery to repair area?
- Is there an open fracture?
- Neurovascular compromise
- Fracture dislocation

Medical History: General

- Past medical or surgical history
- Medications
- Allergies to food or medications
- Family history
- Social history

Medical History: Specific to Complaint

- Family history of musculo-skeletal disease

PHYSICAL EXAMINATION
Vital Signs

- Blood pressure (BP)
- Temperature
- Pulse
- Respiratory rate (RR) and oxygen saturation (SpO_2)

General Appearance
- Amount of distress
- Pain 0/10 and location
- Difficulty with gait or balance

Inspection
- Swelling
- Ecchymosis
- Deformity
- Skin (blisters, abrasions): any open or penetrating wound increases the risk for cellulitis

Palpation
- Area of maximal tenderness
- Tibia
- Fibula
- Fibular neck
- Test for ligament laxity *after acute fracture is ruled out*
- Range of motion (ROM)
- Joint stability

Associated Systems for Assessment
- Dorsalis pedis and posterior tibialis pulses
- Distal capillary refill
- Any indication of vascular compromise: cold, dusky, loss of sensation
- Motor function

CASE STUDY
History

Question	Response
Can you describe what happened when you were injured?	*I was stepping off of the curb and I twisted my ankle*
Can you remember if you stepped on the inside of the ankle or the outside?	*I stepped on the outside of my foot*
Was there pain right away?	*Yes there was; it hurt*
On a scale of 0 to 10 what number would you give the pain?	*Oh, about a 5*
How long did the pain last?	*Well it is still hurting but now it is about a 2 or 3*
Was there immediate swelling?	*Yes, there was, but it has gone down from what it was initially*
Were you able to walk on your foot?	*Yes, I was able to walk to my car okay*
Do you have pain now when you walk on it?	*Yes I do*
Is there any weakness?	*No, not really weak, just pain*
Is there any numbness?	*No there is not*

Question	Response
Have you ever injured your ankle before?	*No*
Do you have any other joint pains?	*No*
Is there any family history of arthritis?	*My mother had it when she was in her 80s*
Do you smoke?	*No*
Do you have any medical illnesses such as diabetes or gout?	*No*
Have you ever taken prednisone or steroids?	*No*

Physical Examination Findings

- VITAL SIGNS: BP 120/80; heart rate (HR) 62; respiratory rate (RR) 18, regular; temperature 98.2°F
- GENERAL APPEARANCE: 48-year-old female, body mass index (BMI) 25, no apparent distress, ambulating to the examination room with a limp, inversion injury
- MUSCULOSKELETAL: lateral ankle anterior talofibular tenderness to palpation, but no pain to posterior edge of medial or lateral malleolus and no midfoot pain; positive swelling present; negative anterior drawer test; talar tilt negative
- SKIN: ecchymosis; skin warm, dry, intact
- EXTREMITIES: distal perfusion intact

Assessing Ankle Injury Severity

Any ankle sprain needs to be assessed as to severity of injury. By using a grade scale the provider can determine the degree of injury and subsequent treatment.

MILD SPRAIN:
- Occurs with slight stretching and minimal damage to the fibers (fibrils) of the ankle ligaments
- Patient can place pressure on foot and walk
- Minimal joint instability
- Mild pain
- Mild swelling
- Some joint stiffness

MODERATE SPRAIN:
- Partial tearing of the ligament
- Abnormal looseness (laxity) of the ankle joint
- Moderate tearing of the ligament fibers
- Some instability of the joint
- Moderate to severe pain and difficulty walking
- Swelling and stiffness
- Minor bruising

SEVERE SPRAIN:
- Complete tear of the ligament occurs
- Total rupture of a ligament
- Gross instability of the joint

- Severe pain initially followed later by no pain
- Severe edema
- Extensive bruising

DIFFERENTIAL DIAGNOSIS

Differential Diagnosis	Fracture or Dislocation: Stable or Unstable	Sprain or Contusion	Achilles Tendonitis
Onset	Abrupt	Abrupt	Abrupt
Bilateral	No	No	No
Deformity	Yes	No	No
Warmth	Yes	Yes	No
Edema	Yes	Yes	No
Skin	Compound fracture	Ecchymosis	Clear intact
Stiffness	No	Yes	Yes
Neurovascular	Yes	Yes	No
Pain	Yes	Yes	Yes

DIAGNOSTIC EXAMINATION

The following tests may reasonably be considered in the initial workup, if indicated.

Examination	Procedure Code	Cost	Results	Notes
Ankle series	73610	$90	Fractures or ligament tears	• Imaging is indicated if the patient has pain in the malleolar zone and bone tenderness at specific sites or experiences the inability to bear weight
Foot series	74022	$100	Fractures	• Imaging is indicated if the patient has midfoot pain and bone tenderness at specific sites or experiences the inability to bear weight immediately

(*continued*)

Examination	Procedure Code	Cost	Results	Notes
MRI	73630	$400 to $3500	Highly effective for early detection and should be ordered early if there is a high level of suspicion for cellulitis, soft tissue abscess, osteomyelitis	• Identifies redundant and inflamed soft tissue • Recommendation is to limit MRI in the ankle ligament for athletes at the advanced competitive level, patients with history of chronic ankle instability, and if suspected deltoid ligament injury
CT	73700	$400 to $3500	Fractures	If suspected fracture of the talus
Bone scan	77080	$200 and $600	Highly effective for early detection and should be ordered early if there is a high level of suspicion for cellulitis, soft tissue abscess, osteomyelitis	Indicated if stress fracture is present; useful for unexplained bone pain, bone infection. injuries undetectable on standard x-ray
MR arthrogram	23350	$1090 and $2339	Talofibular and calcaneal ligament tears, talus defects	• Used to diagnose and for minor intervention to shave away redundant soft tissue and bone • Appropriate for chronic anterior talofibular and calcaneal ligament tears • Osteochondral defect of talus • Anterior ankle impingement due to repetitive stress, usually identified by bone spurs on standard x-ray • Posterior ankle impingement due to overuse • Synovitis, the procedure is used to remove the synovium

CLINICAL DECISION MAKING

Case Study Analysis

The nurse practitioner performs the assessment and physical examination on the patient and finds the following: minor trauma, single site of injury, no neurovascular impairment. Assessment results suggest no indication for imaging at this time.

Diagnosis: Lateral ankle sprain: Mild sprain

Many sports-related traumatic lesions are lateral ankle sprains. The anterior talofibular ligament is the weakest part of the ankle and the most likely area affected by trauma.

BREAST LUMPS

Case Presentation: *A 55-year-old African American social worker presents to your clinic with a finding of a lump in her left breast while in the shower this past week.*

INTRODUCTION TO COMPLAINT

- Family history and other factors can affect a women's perception of this finding
- Several other conditions can cause a breast lump
- All breast lumps need a thorough and systematic approach to history and physical examination

Fibroadenoma

- A fibroadenoma is the most common cause of a breast lump
- It is always benign and made up of a combination of glandular breast tissue and fibroconnective tissue
- Often it can be influenced by hormones and becomes large enough that it is easily felt and sometimes easily visible
- Age as well as definite characteristics will help differentiate the diagnosis of a fibroadenoma as a cause of a breast lump

Cyst

- Cysts are generally fluid filled
- They can be singular or appear in clusters
- Generally, breast cysts decline with menopause and may be present, more frequently, during the luteal phase of a women's menstrual cycle
- Because cysts are influenced by hormones, they may continue to be present in postmenopausal women who are on hormone replacement therapy

Cancer

- Cancer can be another cause of a breast mass
- Often it cannot be diagnosed based on physical examination findings alone
- A breast mass that is a cancer may have characteristics that are a cause for concern but it cannot be diagnosed without a diagnostic evaluation, which will include a biopsy of the mass

HISTORY OF COMPLAINT
Symptomatology

Ask about the following characteristics of each symptom using open-ended questions:

- Onset (sudden or gradual)
- Chronology
- Current situation (improving or deteriorating)
- Location
- Radiation
- Quality
- Timing (frequency, duration)
- Severity
- Precipitating and aggravating factors
- Relieving factors
- Associated symptoms
- Effects on daily activities
- Previous diagnosis of similar episodes
- Previous treatment
- Efficacy of previous treatment

Directed Questions to Ask

The following directed questions will be helpful in collecting the patient's history:

- What was your age of menarche?
- What was your age of menopause (if applicable)?
- Do you have a family history of breast cancer (first-degree relative [mother, sister, or daughter] on either mother's or father's side, age of diagnosis, family history of breast cancer in any male relative)?
- Do you have evidence of breast cancer gene (*BR/CA1/2*)?
- Do you have a personal history of breast cancer?
- What was your age at your first pregnancy?
- Do you use alcohol?
- Do you have a history of chest or neck radiation?
- Do you have a history of breast biopsies and diagnosis?
- Do you use hormones (oral contraceptives or hormone replacement therapy)?
- Are you on a high-fat diet?
- Do you do any physical activities?
- Have there been changes in the lump since initially finding it (size, pain, skin changes, nipple discharge, change with menstrual cycle)?
- Have you had any weight changes, palpable lumps in armpit or under clavicle?

Assessment: Cardinal Signs and Symptoms

In addition to the general characteristics outlined above, additional characteristics of specific symptoms should be elicited as follows:

- General: weight changes, recent fever, chills, general malaise
- Neck and axilla: recent palpable lumps/tenderness
- Breasts: noticeable skin changes, pain, tenderness, nipple discharge
- A complete assessment should include the chest wall, heart, and lungs

Medical History: General

- Relevant past medical conditions and surgeries
- Allergies
- Current medications: prescription, oral contraceptives, hormone replacement, over-the-counter herbal products (dosage and length of treatment)

Medical History: Specific to Complaint

- History of previous breast mass
- Breast biopsy or surgery
- History of ovarian or colon cancer

PHYSICAL EXAMINATION

Vital Signs

- Temperature
- Blood pressure
- Pulse

General Appearance

- Apparent state of health
- Appearance of comfort or distress
- Color, temperature of skin
- General nutritional status
- Hygiene

Neck
- Chest wall
- Axillae
- Supraclavicular, infraclavicular, and axillary adenopathy (sitting and supine)

Breasts
- Visual: sitting and supine
- Observe outline and contour of the breasts: look for any bulging or areas of asymmetry
- Movement of the breasts with arms above the head and at the side, flexion of the pectoral muscles with hands on hips, and pressing in to contract the muscles
- Skin changes: check for dimpling or retraction of the breast tissue, edema, ulceration, erythema or scaling, irritated skin changes, peau d'orange (orange peel appearance)
- Nipples: look for asymmetry, inversion, or retraction; evidence of discharge or crusted exudates

Palpation
- REGIONAL LYMPH NODES: With patient in sitting position, palpate the axillae and infraclavicular and supraclavicular nodes. This is best done with the patient in a relaxed position. Document any findings, observing for position, mobility, tenderness.
- BREAST EXAMINATION: This should be done initially in the sitting position, supporting the breast with one hand and examining with the other. The breasts should then be examined with the patient in the supine position, with the arm on the side you are examining above her head. For a woman with large breasts, it may be helpful for her to roll onto the contralateral hip so that you can better palpate the upper and lower lateral quadrants of the breast you are examining and then complete the examination with her on her back.

The entire breast should be examined using a systematic approach: either using small concentric circles with varying degrees of pressure (light, medium, and deep) or the up and down approach also known as the "lawnmower" method. The finger pads should be used for palpation rather than the fingertips. It is important to cover all breast tissue, imagining a rectangle rather than a circle. Assess for consistency of tissue, presence of tenderness, nodularity, dominant masses, and borders of the mass. Compare asymmetry between breasts.

Documentation
- Document size, shape, borders of a mass. Size should be measured in centimeters, the clock position of the mass should be recorded, and the number of centimeters from the areola should be measured (e.g., 4 × 4 cm circular mass with smooth borders, 10 o'clock position, 5 cm from the nipple)
- Document as much detail as possible, including negative findings

CASE STUDY
History

Question	*Response*
Was the onset sudden or gradual?	*Sudden, found while showering*
Where is the lump located?	*Left breast, upper outer quadrant*
How big is it?	*Feels like a small pea*
Can you move it around?	*No, it doesn't feel like it will move*
Are the borders palpable?	*No, I can't seem to feel the borders easily*
Is there tenderness or pain?	*No, there is no tenderness or pain*
Have you noticed any skin changes or nipple discharge from the left breast?	*No, I have not*
Have you felt any lumps or tenderness in your left armpit?	*No*
When was the last time you had a mammogram?	*Negative screening mammogram 2 years ago*
How old were you when you started to have your periods?	*I was 13 years old*
At what age did you go into menopause?	*I was 52*
Have you ever been pregnant? How old were you when you had your first child?	*I was 26 with my first child*
Did you breastfeed? How long?	*Yes for 4 months*
Did you ever take hormones, either birth control pills or postmenopausal hormone replacement?	*I took birth control pills for 10 years, starting when I was 20* *I am not on hormone replacement*
Have you ever had breast surgeries or a breast biopsy?	*No*

Question	Response
Do you have a family history of breast disease or breast cancer?	*My grandmother had breast cancer when she was 76 years old*
Do you do self-breast exams?	*On occasion*
How has your recent health been?	*Very healthy*
Do you drink alcohol?	*Occasional glass of wine two times a week*
Do you exercise?	*Yes, three to four times a week for 30 minutes*
Do you have a high-fat diet?	*No*

Physical Examination Findings

- VITAL SIGNS: temperature 98.6°F; respiratory rate (RR) 16; heart rate (HR) 80, regular; blood pressure (BP) 120/80; height: 5′8″; weight 160 lbs; body mass index (BMI) 24
- GENERAL APPEARANCE: well developed, nourished, healthy-appearing female
- NECK: supple, no cervical adenopathy
- BREASTS: Examined in sitting and supine positions. In sitting position, no evidence of skin changes, right breast is slightly larger than the left, symmetrical movement with the arms above the head and at the side and with flexion of the pectoral muscles; 5-mm nonmobile, nontender, firm mass felt at 10 o'clock position, 5 cm from the areola. Right breast without dominant masses or tenderness. Nipples without inversion or evidence of nipple discharge. Breast mass is palpated in the supine position in the same manner as in the sitting position
- LYMPH: negative axillary, infraclavicular, and supraclavicular lymphadenopathy
- LUNGS: clear to auscultation
- HEART: regular rate and rhythm (RRR)
- CHEST WALL: symmetrical, no tenderness over intercostals spaces

DIFFERENTIAL DIAGNOSIS

Differential Diagnosis	Cyst	Fibroadenoma	Cancer
Onset	Sudden	Gradual	Gradual/sudden
Age	15–55	15–25 (puberty/young adult)	30–90: more common >50, postmenopause
Cyclic	Can be cyclic	Usually not	Not related
Hormone influenced	Can be	Can be	Can be/but not caused by
Shape	Round or elongated	Round or elongated	Irregular
Borders	Well defined	Smooth, well defined	Difficult to define
Tenderness	Usually tender	Nontender	Nontender

(continued)

Differential Diagnosis	Cyst	Fibroadenoma	Cancer
Skin changes	Not present	Not present	May be present; peau d'orange
Nipple discharge	Not present	Not present	Usually not present
Mobility	Mobile	Very mobile	Nonmobile, may be fixed to chest wall

DIAGNOSTIC EXAMINATION

Examination	Procedure Code	Cost*	Diagnostic Breast Imaging
Mammogram	77055	$385	Mammogram
		$75 to $100	Radiology fee
Ultrasound	76645	$279	Ultrasound
		$50 to $75	Radiology fee

*These are approximate fees that may vary by facility and region.

CLINICAL DECISION MAKING

Case Study Analysis

The advanced practice nurse (APN) performs the assessment and physical examination on the patient and finds the following data: Sudden onset of a lump in the upper outer quadrant of the left breast found while in the shower. It is nontender and nonmobile. There are no skin changes or evidence of nipple discharge. She has no other symptoms. She cannot feel any lumps under her arm or under her collarbone. She has never had a positive-screening mammogram, nor does she have a history of breast biopsies or surgeries. She is menopausal and not currently taking hormone replacement. She has a family history of a maternal grandmother with breast cancer diagnosed in her 70s. She is worried and concerned as a coworker was recently diagnosed with breast cancer. Her physical examination reveals a 5-mm size firm, nonmobile mass at 10 o'clock position in the left breast, 5 cm from the nipple. There is negative lymphadenopathy.

> *Diagnosis:* Pending mammogram results

In women under 30 this will include a unilateral breast ultrasound and in women over 30 a diagnostic mammogram and ultrasound.

It should never be assumed by the clinician that a diagnosis can be made based on the history and physical examination alone. In young women, it may be advisable to observe the breast lump over a menstrual cycle to see if there are changes, especially if tenderness is a symptom and the lump is found during the luteal phase of the menstrual cycle.

A negative clinical examination is not conclusive of a negative diagnosis of cancer even in light of a negative mammogram and ultrasound. All palpable lumps with negative imaging should be referred to a breast surgeon for final diagnosis and management.

CHEST PAIN

Case Presentation: *A 70-year-old female reports experiencing pain in her chest while walking up steps today.*

INTRODUCTION TO COMPLAINT

Chest pain can be caused by several serious, life-threatening disorders, such as cardiac ischemia, pulmonary embolus, or pneumonia. However, chest pain is a common complaint and may also be caused by non-life-threatening problems, such as arthritis, acid reflux, or panic disorder.

Cardiac Chest Pain

- Chest pain triggered by exertion, eating a meal, emotional distress; is relieved with rest
- Usual risk factors for coronary disease are present, such as hypertension, diabetes, or hyperlipidemia
- Pericarditis, or inflammation of the sac around the heart, causes chest pain that becomes worse when lying down and is relieved when leaning forward

Pulmonary

- Chest pain that increases with a deep breath is termed pleuritic chest pain
- It is usually sharp, stabbing, and associated with inflammation of the pleural lining
- It is associated with pneumonia, pulmonary embolus (PE), autoimmune disease, and viral infections

Musculoskeletal

- Pain in the joints of the costochondral junction is common with increased movement
- It is always reproducible by movement or pressure

Gastrointestinal

- Acid reflux can cause a burning pain or spasm in the midchest and mimics cardiac pain
- It may be precipitated by eating a fatty meal and then lying down, especially if obese
- It is relieved with antacids or acid blockers

Clinical Pearls
- Exertional chest pain relieved with rest strongly suggests ischemic heart disease
- Pleuritic chest pain with shortness of breath indicates a pulmonary embolus or pneumonia
- Musculoskeletal pain is always reproducible with motion or direct pressure over the painful area

HISTORY OF COMPLAINT

Symptomatology

Ask about the following characteristics of each symptom using open-ended questions:

- Onset: Did it come on suddenly or gradually?
- Location/radiation: Can you put a finger on the pain and show me where it goes?
- Duration, timing: How long has the pain been there? Does it come and go? Is it there now?
- Characteristics of the pain: Can you describe, in your own words, how the pain feels?
- Associated symptoms: Did you notice any other symptoms when you had the pain?
- Aggravating factors: Did anything trigger the pain or make it worse?
- Alleviating factors: Did anything relieve the pain, or make it better?
- Effect on daily activities: Has this pain affected your daily activities?

Directed Questions to Ask

- Is the pain worse with exertion?
- Is it relieved with rest?
- Does the pain radiate to the neck, jaw, or arm?
- Is the pain worse with a deep breath?
- Are you having difficulty breathing because of the pain?
- Does movement make the pain worse?
- Have you had heartburn?
- Is the pain worse after eating a meal?
- Is the pain worse when lying down? If so, is it better when sitting up or leaning forward?
- Have you had this pain in the past?
- If so, how did you treat it?

Assessment: Cardinal Signs and Symptoms

The following signs and symptoms are highly associated with some types of chest pain.

Symptom and Signs	Disorder
Constitutional	
Fever, chills, and sweats	Pneumonia, pericarditis
Respiratory	
Chest pain with deep breath	Pleurisy, pulmonary embolus, pneumonia

(*continued*)

Symptom and Signs	Disorder
Shortness of breath	Pneumonia, pulmonary embolus (PE), cardiac disease, congestive heart failure (CHF)
Cardiovascular	
Hypertension, high cholesterol, diabetes	Ischemic heart disease
Exertional chest pain relieved with rest	Ischemic heart disease, valvular heart disease
Palpitation	Cardiac arrhythmia
Gastrointestinal	
Heartburn or acid reflux	Gastroesophageal reflux disease (GERD), esophageal spasm, atypical ischemia
Nausea, vomiting	Ischemic heart disease, GERD, or peptic ulcer
Vascular	
Swelling of both lower extremities	CHF
Swelling of one lower extremity	Deep vein thrombosis (DVT) and subsequent pulmonary embolus
Skin	
Cyanosis	Pneumonia, ischemic heart disease, chronic obstructive pulmonary disease (COPD)
Clubbing of nails	COPD, lung cancer

Medical History: General

- Past medical conditions: ask about history of high cholesterol, smoking, hypertension, type 2 diabetes, other chronic illness
- Medications: Is the patient taking aspirin, nitroglycerin, a nonsteroidal anti-inflammatory drug (NSAID), or any new drug?
- Family history: ask about family history of early heart disease, stroke, transient ischemic attack (TIA), diabetes, high cholesterol, or sudden death
- Social history: ask about occupation, stressors, habits such as smoking, alcohol, exercise, diet habits

PHYSICAL EXAMINATION

Vital Signs

- Temperature/pulse/respiration (TPR)
- Blood pressure (BP)
- Pulse oximetry

General Appearance

- Does the patient appear to be in acute distress, fearful, diaphoretic? Is there obvious shortness of breath?
- Does the patient appear to be healthy and relaxed?

Neck

- Palpate carotid arteries for symmetry of stroke and listen for bruit
- Evaluate the jugular venous pressure at a 45-degree angle

Cardiopulmonary

HEART:
- Listen for S1 and S2 and identify any abnormal sounds, such as a murmur, gallop, or friction rub
- Palpate the point of maximum impulse (PMI)
- Determine whether rhythm is regular or irregular
- Count the heart rate if it is excessively slow or rapid

LUNGS:
- Observe character of respiration and confirm whether labored, rapid, shallow
- Listen for quality of breath sounds: are they clear, diminished, or absent?
- Listen for adventitious sounds, such as crackles (rales), rhonchi, or friction rubs
- Percuss the chest to identify dullness indicating pleural effusion or pneumonia
- Perform E to A testing. If there is a consolidation, when the patient says "E" it will sound like an "A." Tactile fremitus is increased if there is a lobar pneumonia. If there is dullness to percussion, this indicates fluid rather than air in the lungs.

Abdomen

- Observe the abdominal aorta for abnormally wide or prominent pulsations
- Listen to the abdomen for bowel tones and bruits
- Percuss the abdomen to identify areas of tympany, dullness, or tenderness
- Palpate the abdomen to identify areas of tenderness, organomegaly, or masses

Vascular/Extremities

- Observe lower extremities for edema, check capillary refill and distal pulses

Skin

- Observe for pallor or cyanosis
- Check nails for clubbing or cyanosis of nail bed

Neurological

- Describe mental status
- Is the patient alert and oriented or confused and somnolent?

CASE STUDY

History

A 70-year-old female presents to the urgent care walk-in clinic stating that she woke up at about 3 a.m. with pain in the center of her chest. It went away after a few hours, but was there when she woke up in the morning. She reports no shortness of breath, diaphoresis, or fatigue. She has not had fever or chills.

Question	*Response*
Are you having the discomfort right now?	*Yes, but very little now*
Can you describe it?	*It is like an ache or a burning sensation*
Where is it? Can you put a finger on it?	*Yes, right here (center of sternum)*
Does it go anywhere else in the chest?	*Up into my throat*
Does it go into the arms at all?	*No, my arms feel fine*
On a scale of 0 to 10, what was it?	*Oh, I'd say an 8 or so*
What is it now?	*Oh, a 2 or so*
Does anything make it worse?	*Yes, I couldn't sleep last night*
Was the pain worse when you were lying down?	*Oh yes, much worse*
Did anything make it better?	*Yes, sitting up helped*
Did anything else help?	*Yes, drinking a glass of water*
Was it worse when you walked around today?	*No, can't say it was*
Was it worse going up steps?	*No, it wasn't*
Did you feel weak or sweaty with the pain?	*Yes, a little bit*
Did you feel nauseated?	*Yes, a little bit*
Did you vomit?	*No, I didn't*
Do you have a history of a stomach ulcer?	*No, I never have*
Do you have a history of acid reflux?	*No, I never have that I know of*
Do you have high blood pressure?	*Yes, I take medication for it*
What is the name of the medication?	*Procardia, I just started this new one*
Do you have high cholesterol?	*No, my doctor said that is fine*
Do you have heart disease, like angina?	*No, I don't think so*
Do you ever have to stop what you are doing due to chest pain, pressure, nausea, or heartburn?	*No, I never have had to do that*
Does your heart ever race fast, or beat irregularly?	*Not that I have ever noticed*
Do your legs ever swell up?	*No, they don't do that*
Do you feel short of breath?	*No, I breathe just fine*
Does the pain feel worse when you take in a deep breath?	*(takes deep breath) No, it doesn't*
Does it hurt when you press on the chest?	*(presses) No, it doesn't*
What did you eat last night before bed?	*Mexican food, chips, and salsa*

Physical Examination Findings

- VITAL SIGNS: BP 129/70, heart rate (HR) 72 and regular, respiratory rate (RR) 16 unlabored, temperature 98.8°F, oral pulse oximetry is 99%
- GENERAL APPEARANCE: pleasant obese female, alert, in no acute distress.
- SKIN: warm, dry, color is normal
- NECK: carotids are 2+ without bruits; thyroid is not palpable; no lymphadenopathy
- HEART: S1 and S2 normal without murmur, gallop, or rub
- LUNGS: clear and resonant
- CHEST WALL: nontender along the sternal border and rib areas
- ABDOMEN: bowel tones are normal, no abdominal bruit; abdomen is soft, slightly tender in the epigastric area, no masses or organomegaly
- RECTAL: rectal vault nontender; stool is negative for blood
- EXTREMITIES: radial and pedal pulses 2+ and equal; no edema, cyanosis, or clubbing of the nails

DIFFERENTIAL DIAGNOSIS

Diagnosis	History	Physical Examination	Diagnostic Tests
Angina	Triggered by exertion and relieved by rest in < 30 minutes	Often normal; listen for S3, S4, or murmurs; or abnormal BP	EKG, stress test, lipid panel, cardiac enzymes
Acute coronary syndrome	Substernal, radiates to neck, jaw, lasts > 30 minutes, diaphoretic, nausea, vomiting	Pale, sweaty; may have S3, S4, rales, murmur; or normal examination	EKG, troponin, creatinine kinase isoenzyme MB (CK-MB), coronary angiogram
Pericarditis	Chest pain that is stabbing, worse lying down, better leaning forward	Hallmark is pericardial friction rub; increased jugular venous pressure (JVP) or edema lower extremities (LE)	EKG, chest x-ray (CXR), echo, MRI, pericardial tap, high erythrocyte sedimentation rate (ESR), plus blood cultures or plus antinuclear antibodies (ANA)
Pleuritic	Pain worse with deep respirations	Pleural friction rub	CXR or EKG, complete blood count (CBC), ESR, ANA, D-dimer
Pneumonia	Fever, cough	Crackles over lobe	Chest x-ray, CBC/white blood count (WBC)
Pulmonary embolism	Dyspnea, pleuritic pain, leg swelling, calf pain, risk factors	Rapid RR, and HR, pleural friction rub, unilateral edema LE	CT angiography or ventilation/ perfusion (V/Q) scan, arterial blood gases (ABGs), D-dimer, venous doppler
Pneumothorax	Sudden dyspnea running or trauma	Decreased or absent breath sounds	Chest x-ray shows loss of lung markings
Musculoskeletal	Worst with motion or pressure to local area	Pain reproducible	Physical examination

(continued)

Diagnosis	History	Physical Examination	Diagnostic Tests
GERD/ esophageal	Pain lying down, after eating fatty meal	Better sitting up or with antacid/lidocaine	Endoscopy or upper gastrointestinal scan (GI)
Aortic dissection	M:F 3:1; age 60 to 80; sudden onset of severe, sharp chest pain radiating into back, syncope	Severe hypertension; >20 mmHg in BP between arms; absent distal pulses; early manifestations: Horner's syndrome, sudden hoarseness	EKG to rule out myocardial infarction (MI); chest x-ray, transesophageal echo (TEE), MRI, and helical CT are options

DIAGNOSTIC EXAMINATION

Examination	Procedure Code	Cost	Indication and Interpretation
Electrocardiogram	93000	$150	If cardiac risk factors are present, exertional chest pain may reveal classic changes of ischemia; a normal EKG does not rule out ischemia
Cardiac troponins	84484	$300	Elevated in ischemic as well as other cardiac disease
CK-MB isoenzymes	82553	$300	Evidence of ischemic heart disease
Beta natriuretic peptide (BNP)	83880	$250	Secreted by ventricles in response to volume overload in CHF, high in renal failure
CBC	85025	$75	Identifies anemia or elevated WBC
Comprehensive metabolic panel	83516	$120	Evaluates electrolytes, renal and liver status

DIAGNOSTIC IMAGING TESTS

Examination	Procedure Code	Cost	Indications and Interpretation
Chest x-ray	71020	$250	Shortness of breath, fever, ischemic or pleuritic chest pain; may reveal pulmonary congestion from CHF, pneumonia, pleural thickening, or effusion
Cardiac echo	93351	$1500	Evaluate patients with ischemic heart disease for structural abnormalities, abnormal wall motion abnormal valves, and ejection fraction
Stress testing	93015	$800	If cardiac chest pain is present, exercise treadmill, stress echo, or radionuclide testing

(*continued*)

Examination	Procedure Code	Cost	Indications and Interpretation
Coronary angiography	75574	$2500	Invasive but gold standard for ruling in or ruling out the presence of coronary artery disease (CAD)
CT spiral	74000	$1200	If a pulmonary embolus is suspected due to sudden shortness of breath
Chest CT	71275	$1800	If aortic dissection, pneumonia, effusion are suspected

Basic Interpretation of EKG

T wave inversion, ST segment elevation, or Q waves are diagnostic of an ST elevation MI (STEMI), indicating damage through the entire wall of the ventricle. The leads that are abnormal indicate the area of cardiac injury. "Q waves" develop over 12 to 16 hours and indicate an older cardiac injury.

EKG Leads	Ischemic Area of Heart
V1 through V6	Anterior or anterolateral
Leads I and aVL	Lateral
Leads II, III, and augmented voltage foot (AVF)	Inferior
No cardiac changes	No ischemia or non-STEMI

Diagnostic testing reveals the following:

- EKG, troponins, CK-MB, CBC, renal and liver studies are normal
- Echocardiogram reveals no abnormalities

CLINICAL DECISION MAKING

Case Study Analysis

A 70-year-old female who, after eating a fatty, spicy meal, wakes up at 3 a.m. with substernal chest pain associated with burning in the chest that was relieved on sitting up and also on taking antacids. Her pertinent negatives are the absence of exertional chest pain, dyspnea, lower extremity edema. She started taking a new medication "Procardia," which can cause relaxation of the lower esophageal sphincter, leading to acid reflux and esophageal spasm. Her differential diagnosis includes atypical chest pain, cardiac ischemia, or gastric acid reflux. Her cardiac enzymes, EKG, and echo are normal.

> **Diagnosis:** *Likely side effect of new medication "Procardia," which can cause relaxation of the lower esophageal sphincter, leading to acid reflux and esophageal spasm.*

FURTHER READING

Ferri, F. F. (2010). *Ferri's best test* (2nd ed.). Philadelphia, PA: Elsevier Mosby.

Ferri, F. F. (2011). *Ferri's clinical advisor*. Philadelphia, PA: Elsevier Mosby.

McConaghy, J. R., & Oza, R. S. (2013). Outpatient diagnosis of acute chest pain in adults. *American Family Physician, 87*(3), 177–182.

McGee, S. (2007). *Evidence-based physical diagnosis* (2nd ed.). St. Louis, MO: Saunders.

Paauw, D. S., Migeon, M. B., & Burkholder, L. R. (2003). *Internal medicine clerkship guide* (2nd ed.). St. Louis, MO: Mosby.

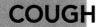

COUGH

Case Presentation: *A 75-year-old female with chronic obstructive pulmonary disease (COPD) presents to the clinic with a cough she has had for the past 2 weeks.*

INTRODUCTION TO COMPLAINT

A cough is the body's natural response to stimuli that irritate the larynx, trachea, and large bronchi. It can be caused by a problem in the upper and lower airways, disruptions in the cardiovascular system, and side effects from certain medications. It is the fifth most common symptom prompting physician visits.

Acute Cough

Cough that lasts less than 3 weeks.

- Viral rhinosinusitis
- Viral bronchitis
- Postnasal drip due to allergy or sinus disease
- COPD or asthma exacerbation
- Pneumonia

Chronic Cough

Cough that lasts longer than 8 weeks.

- Chronic bronchitis
- Postnasal drip
- Airway hyperresponsiveness after resolution of a viral or bacterial respiratory infection (i.e., postinfection cough)
- Asthma
- Medications, especially angiotensin converting enzyme (ACE) inhibitors
- Gastroesophageal reflux

Red Flags
The following findings are of particular concern:

- Dyspnea
- Hemoptysis
- Weight loss
- Risk factors for tuberculosis (TB) or HIV infection
- Wheezing
- Fever, night sweats, and weight loss

Allergies

- Dust
- Smoke
- Pollen or mold
- Pets
- Plants
- Cleaning agents and room deodorizers
- Chemical fumes
- Postnasal drip caused by allergies

Medicines

- ACE chronic cough

Other Causes

- Compression in air passage from a tumor
- Enlarged peribronchial lymph nodes
- Impacted cerumen or a foreign body in the external auditory canal triggers reflex cough through stimulation of the auricular branch of the vagus nerve
- Pulmonary embolism

HISTORY OF COMPLAINT

Symptomatology

Ask about the following characteristics of each symptom using open-ended questions:

- Current situation (improving or deteriorating)
- Onset (acute or gradual)
- Characteristics of the cough (i.e., whether dry or producing sputum or blood)
- Associated symptoms
- Aggravating factors or triggers
- Alleviating factors
- Effect on daily activities

Directed Questions to Ask

- What time does the cough occur (i.e., primarily at night)?
- Do you have any shortness of breath?
- Do you have difficulty swallowing?
- Do you have pain with swallowing?
- Do you have a sore throat?
- Do you have heartburn?
- Do you have the need to clear your throat frequently? Postnasal drainage?
- Is it worse at night when lying down?
- Are there any precipitating factors (i.e., cold air, strong odors)?
- Do you experience any pain with your cough? When and where is the pain?
- Are you coughing up phlegm?
- Is the cough dry, brassy, or high pitched and unproductive?
- Are you wheezing (making a whistling sound when you breathe)?
- Are you feeling feverish? Have you taken your temperature?

- Are you losing weight without trying?
- Are you having drenching sweats in bed at night?
  (the sheets and your pajamas get soaking wet)
- Does anything relieve your cough?
- Does anything trigger your cough, such as running, talking, or laughing?
- Are there any other associated symptoms?
- How does the cough affect your daily activities?
- Have you had a previous diagnosis of similar episodes?
- Have you had previous treatments for your cough?
- What medications do you take?
- Do you have a history of allergies?
- Do you smoke? If so, how many packs per year?
- Do you drink alcohol?
- Do you have family members who have a cough now or in the past?

Assessment: Cardinal Signs and Symptoms

In addition to the general characteristics outlined above, additional characteristics of specific symptoms should be elicited, as follows:

Constitutional
- Fever
- Chills
- Sweats
- Malaise
- Weight loss

Eyes
- Itching, watery

Ears
- Pain
- Drainage
- Hearing loss

Nose/Oropharynx
- Cobblestone appearance (postnasal drainage)
- Runny nose

Sinuses
- Palpate
- Percuss
- Transilluminate

Mouth/Throat/Pharynx
- Pale
- Boggy
- Swollen
- Difficulty swallowing
- Choking episodes while eating or drinking (aspiration)
- Sore throat (upper respiratory infection [URI], postnasal drip)

Neck
- Pain
- Swelling
- Enlarged lymph nodes

Trachea/Larynx
- Inspiratory strider

Lungs
- Hyperresonant on percussion
- Distant breath sounds, scattered rhonchi, or wheezing on auscultation
- Prolonged expiration
- Bilateral expiratory wheezes
- Unilateral wheezing
- Basilar rales
- Crackles
- Rales
- Pleuritic chest pain

Cardiovascular System
- Edema or weight loss (tumor, TB)
- Tachycardia
- Gallop

Gastrointestinal
- Heartburn (gastroesophageal reflux)

Skin
- Color
- Temperature
- Turgor
- Capillary refill response

Other Associated Symptoms
- Night sweats
- Fever
- Chills

Medical History: General
- History of allergies
- Smoking history
- Drug history (should specifically include use of ACE inhibitors)
- Past surgical history
- Past medical history

Medical History: Specific to Complaint
- Recent respiratory infections (i.e., within previous 1–2 months)
- Asthma
- COPD
- Gastroesophageal reflux disease

- Exposure to TB
- HIV infection
- Exposure to potential respiratory irritants
- Exposure to known allergens
- Travel to regions with endemic fungal illnesses

PHYSICAL EXAMINATION

Note: If the patient is coughing during the examination, document character and frequency.

Vital Signs

- Respiratory rate
- Fever
- Pulse rate
- Oxygen saturation (SpO_2)
- Blood pressure

General Appearance

- Apparent state of health
- Appearance of comfort or distress
- Skin color
- Nutritional status
- State of hydration
- Hygiene
- Match between appearance and stated age
- Difficulty with gait or balance
- Signs of respiratory distress
- Chronic illness (i.e., wasting, lethargy)

Inspection

Nose and Throat
- Focus on appearance of the nasal mucosa (i.e., color, congestion)
- Presence of discharge (external or in posterior pharynx)
- Drainage, redness, and edema
- Illuminate sinuses
- Swollen tonsils
- Exudate on tonsils

Ears
- Exam for triggers of reflex cough

Neck Inspection
- Symmetry
- Swelling
- Masses
- Active range of motion
- Thyroid enlargement
- Swallowing

- Tracheal deviation
- Cervical and supraclavicular areas inspected and palpated for lymphadenopathy

Lung Examination
- Adequacy of air entry and exit
- Symmetry of breath sounds
- Presence of crackles, wheezes, or both
- Signs of consolidation (e.g., egophony, dullness to percussion)

Cardiovascular
- Pulse strength
- Murmurs
- S1 S2
- S3 S4, gallop, pericardial effusion, muffled heart tones

CASE STUDY
History

Question	Response
When did the symptoms start?	*Started about 2 weeks ago*
Did the cough start suddenly or was it gradual over time?	*Did not pay much attention to it, husband noticed*
What time does the cough occur (i.e., primarily at night)?	*Worse at night*
Do you have any shortness of breath?	*Yes, I feel short of breath*
Do you have difficulty swallowing?	*No*
Do you have pain with swallowing?	*No*
Do you have a sore throat?	*No*
Do you have heartburn?	*No*
Do you have the need to clear your throat frequently?	*No*
Is it worse at night when lying down?	*No*
Are there any precipitating factors (i.e., cold air, strong odors)?	*No*
Are you coughing up anything?	*Yes, yellow-green stuff*
Do you experience any pain with your cough?	*No*
Are you wheezing (making a whistling sound when you breathe)?	*No*
Are you running a temperature?	*Yes, I didn't take it, I feel hot*

Question	Response
Are you having drenching sweats in bed at night? (the sheets and your pajamas get soaking wet)	*Yes, the past 3 days*
Does anything relieve your cough?	*Cough drops, but they don't help*
Are there any other associated symptoms?	*I feel very weak and tired*
How does the cough affect your daily activities?	*Yes, I just can't do much*
Have you had a previous diagnosis of similar episodes?	*No*
Have you had previous treatments for your cough?	*Just the cough drops*
What medications do you take?	*A water pill for blood pressure*
Do you have a history of allergies?	*No, I never had allergies*
Do you smoke? If so, how many packs per year?	*No I do not, husband smokes outside of house*
Do you drink alcohol?	*Social, a glass of wine occasionally*
Do you have family members who have a cough now or in the past?	*No*

Physical Examination Findings

- VITAL SIGNS: temperature 102°F, blood pressure (BP) 120/88, heart rate (HR) 120, respiratory rate (RR) 30
- GENERAL APPEARANCE: patient appears tired; skin color pale, patient diaphoretic and sweaty, short stature, and overweight; height 5′4″; weight 170 lbs
- EARS: no drainage, no tenderness
- EYES: no drainage; pupils equal, round, and reactive to light and accommodation (PERRLA)
- NOSE: clear nasal discharge, turbinates clear, nares clear, nasal sinuses clear, no septum deviation, mucus pink not boggy, and no tenderness
- MOUTH: no oral lesions; membranes dry; teeth and gums in good repair
- PHARYNX: Posterior pharynx without redness or postnasal drip; tonsils absent
- NECK: no lymphadenopathy in any nodes; no other cervical nodes palpable; neck is supple; thyroid is not enlarged
- CHEST: lung crackles left lower base without wheezes or rhonchi; do not clear with coughing; dullness to percussion over the left lower lobe (LLL); RR is 30, shallow, no use of accessory muscles
- ABDOMEN: soft, round, nontender; no organomegaly or masses
- SKIN: skin color pale, warm, and moist; no rashes
- EXTREMITIES: no clubbing, cyanosis, or edema

DIFFERENTIAL DIAGNOSIS

Differential Diagnosis	Sore Throat	Fever	Productive Cough	Dyspnea	Head-ache	Chest Pain	Weight Loss	Hemo-ptysis	Dry Cough	Night Sweat
URI (including acute bronchitis)	Yes	Low	Yes or no	Mild	Yes or no	No	No	No	Yes	No
Pneumonia (viral, bacterial, aspiration, rarely fungal)	Rare	Yes, high	Yes or no	Yes	Yes or no	Yes or no	No	Yes or no	Yes or no	Yes
Postnasal drip (allergic, bacterial origin)	Yes scratchy	No	No	No	Yes or no	No	No	No	Yes	No
COPD exacerbation	No	No	Yes or no	Yes	No	No	No	No	Yes or no	No
Pulmonary embolism (PE)	No	No	Yes or no	Yes, severe	No	Yes with deep breath	No	Occa-sional	Yes	No
Asthma	No	No	No	Yes	No	No	No	No	Yes	No
ACE inhibitors	No	No	No	No	No	No	No	No	Yes	No
Tumor	No	Yes or no	Yes or no	No	No	Yes or no	No	Yes or no	Yes	Yes or no
TB or fungal infections	No	Yes	No	No	No	No	Yes	Yes	No	Yes or no

DIAGNOSTIC EXAMINATION

Examination	Procedure Code	Cost	Results
Chest radiography (x-ray)	71020	$300	• Shows heart, lungs, airway, blood vessels, and lymph nodes • Bones of spine and chest, including breastbone, ribs, collarbone, and the upper part of spine • The most common imaging test or x-ray used to find pathology
CT scan thorax with contrast (testing to be performed only if positive chest x-ray and high suspicion for PE or lung cancer)	71260	$1400	Cross-sectional images of a part of the body are formed through computerized axial tomography and shown on a computer screen
Complete blood count (CBC)	85025	$75	The CBC typically has several parameters. These are the most relevant: White blood count (WBC) • High WBC can be a sign of infection • WBC is also increased in certain types of leukemia • Decreased WBCs can be a sign of bone marrow diseases or an enlarged spleen or HIV Hemoglobin (Hgb) and hematocrit (Hct) • Hgb is the amount of oxygen-carrying protein contained within the red blood cells (RBCs) • Hct is the percentage of the blood volume occupied by RBCs • Low Hgb or Hct suggests an anemia • High Hgb can occur due to lung disease, living at high altitudes, or excessive bone marrow production of blood cells MCV • This helps diagnose a cause of anemia; low values suggest iron deficiency; high values suggest deficiencies of either vitamin B_{12} or folate, ineffective production in the bone marrow, or recent blood loss with replacement by newer (and larger) cells from the bone marrow Platelet count • High values can occur with bleeding, cigarette smoking; low values can occur from premature destruction or excess production by the bone marrow • States such as immune thrombocytopenia, acute blood loss, drug effects (such as heparin), infections with sepsis, entrapment of platelets in an enlarged spleen, or bone marrow failure from diseases such as myelofibrosis or leukemia

(continued)

Examination	Procedure Code	Cost	Results
TB skin test (testing to be performed only if high suspicion for TB)	86580	$20	The TB skin test is used to determine whether someone has developed an immune response to the bacterium that causes TB; this response can occur if someone currently has TB, if he or she was exposed to it in the past, or if he or she received the Bacille Calmette Guerin (BCG) vaccine against TB Negative: Induration of < 2 mm Positive: Induration > 15 mm normal immune system, > 10 mm induration health care worker or personal contact of someone with active TB, > 5 mm induration immunocompromised
D-dimer (testing to be performed only if there is high suspicion for PE)	85379	$80	A normal or negative D-dimer result means that it is most likely that the person tested does not have an acute condition or disease that is causing abnormal clot formation and breakdown A positive D-dimer result may indicate the presence of an abnormally high level of fibrin degradation products. It tells the doctor that there may be significant blood clot (thrombus) formation and breakdown in the body
EKG (testing to be performed only if high suspicion of cough related to cardiac causes, such as congestive heart failure [CHF])	93000	$800	An EKG is used to measure: • Any damage to the heart • How fast your heart is beating and whether it is beating normally • The effects of drugs or devices used to control the heart (such as a pacemaker) • The size and position of your heart chambers • Normal heart rate: 60 to 100 beats per minute • Heart rhythm: consistent and even Abnormal EKG results may be a sign of: • Abnormal heart rhythms (arrhythmias) • Damage or changes to the heart muscle • Changes in the amount of sodium or potassium in the blood • Congenital heart defect • Enlargement of the heart • Fluid or swelling in the sac around the heart • Inflammation of the heart (myocarditis) • Past or current heart attack
Pulse oximetry	94760	$15	Oximetry measures the concentration of oxygen in the blood; the test is used for the evaluation of various medical conditions that affect the function of the heart and lungs Normal results: between 95% and 100% at room temperature Low normal: 90% to 95% at room temperature Abnormal results: below 90% at room temperature

Examination	Procedure Code	Cost	Results
Bronchoscopy (testing to be performed only if high suspicion for lung cancer)	31622	$800	Bronchoscopy is a procedure that allows the doctor to look at the patient's airway through a thin viewing instrument called a bronchoscope Bronchoscopy may be done either to diagnose problems with the airway, the lungs, or the lymph nodes in the chest or to treat problems such as an object or growth in the airway

CLINICAL DECISION MAKING

Case Study Analysis

Rapid heart and respiratory rate with presence of fever indicate the need for a chest x-ray, which confirms left lower lobe pneumonia, and CBC shows WBC 20,000. Pertinent negatives are hemoptysis, weight loss, sinus pain, nasal discharge, wheezes, and rhonchi.

Diagnosis: Left lower lobe pneumonia

DIARRHEA

Case Presentation: *A 37-year-old European American female presents to your practice with "loose stools."*

INTRODUCTION TO COMPLAINT
Definition of Diarrhea

Diarrhea is a common manifestation of a number of gastrointestinal (GI) diseases. The definition is based on the frequency, *volume*, and consistency of stools. The patient's perception of the stool and the components of a definition of diarrhea often are variable.

- Acute: lasting less than 14 days in duration
- Persistent: more than 14 days in duration
- Chronic: more than 30 days in duration

Chronic diarrhea involves a decrease in stool consistency of more than 1 month duration.

Etiology for Acute Diarrhea
- VIRAL: most common; examples of viruses are norovirus, adenovirus, rotovirus
- BACTERIAL: usually severe but self-limiting; examples of bacteria are *Salmonella, Shigella, Staphylococcus aureus, Clostridium difficile, Campylobacter*
- PROTOZOAL: not usually identified as a cause of diarrhea in the developed world; examples of protozoa are *Giardia lamblia, Cryptosporidium, Entamoeba histolytica*

Etiology for Chronic Diarrhea
- IRRITABLE BOWEL SYNDROME (IBS): defined as a symptom complex of chronic lower abdominal pain; altered bowel habits are the primary characteristic of IBS
- FUNCTIONAL DIARRHEA: defined as continuous or recurrent passage of loose (mushy) or watery stools with abdominal pain or discomfort
- INFLAMMATORY BOWEL DISEASE (IBD): refers primarily to Crohn's disease and ulcerative colitis; Crohn's disease may involve the entire GI tract; ulcerative colitis is often defined as mild, moderate, or severe and often presents in a variable manner with diarrhea as its main symptom
- MICROSCOPIC COLITIS: seen as chronic watery (secretory) diarrhea without bleeding; usually occurs in middle-aged patients but can affect children
- MALABSORPTION SYNDROME: is defined as impaired absorption of nutrients; it occurs as a result of congenital defects in the transport system, acquired defects, such as celiac disease, extensive surgical resection (gastric bypass)
- CHOLECYSTECTOMY: diarrhea occurs in 5% to 12% of patients; it will resolve or improve over the course of weeks to months and is related to excessive bile acids entering the colon

- CHRONIC INFECTIONS: persistent bacterial and protozoal infections can be seen in patients with chronic diarrhea; specific risk factors should be assessed such as travel, HIV infection, use of antibiotics, and consumption of contaminated drinking water

HISTORY OF COMPLAINT

Symptomatology

Ask about the following characteristics of each symptom using open-ended questions:

- Onset (sudden or gradual)
- Chronology
- Current situation (improving or deteriorating)
- Location
- Radiation
- Quality
- Timing (frequency, duration)
- Severity
- Precipitating and aggravating factors
- Relieving factors
- Associated symptoms
- Effects on daily activities
- Previous diagnosis of similar episodes
- Previous treatments
- Efficacy of previous treatments

Directed Questions to Ask

- How long have you had diarrhea?
- How frequently have you had diarrhea?
- Can you describe the color and consistency?
- Any associated symptoms? Fever? Abdominal pain? Nausea/vomiting?
- Where do you live/reside? Facility?
- What is your occupation?
- Any particular hobbies?
- Have you traveled anywhere recently?
- Have you traveled anywhere in the past year?
- What have you eaten in the past 24 hours, past 48 hours?
- Have you been on antibiotics recently?

Assessment: Cardinal Signs and Symptoms

In addition to the general characteristics outlined above, additional characteristics of specific symptoms should be elicited as follows:

General
- Fever, chills, malaise
- Fatigue
- Night sweats
- Weight, diet

Throat and Mouth

- Hoarseness
- Sore throat
- Ulcers
- Bleeding
- Teeth
- Taste

GI

- Heartburn
- Constipation
- Pain
- Appetite
- Blood
- Flatulence
- Hemorrhoids
- Jaundice
- Normal stool color

Medical History: General

- Medical conditions and surgeries
- Allergies (seasonal and others)
- Medication currently used (prescription, birth control pill [BCP] and over the counter [OTC])
- Herbal preparations and traditional therapies

Medical History: Specific to Complaint

- Risk factor for HIV infection
- Recent weight loss
- Fecal incontinence
- Fevers, joint pains, mouth ulcers, eye redness
- Family history specific to IBD
- Medications

Medical History: Specific to GI System

- Chronic GI disorders
- GI surgeries
- Trauma
- For other specific questions related to chronic diarrhea, see above

PHYSICAL EXAMINATION

Vital Signs

- Temperature
- Pulse
- Respiration
- SpO_2 (oxygen saturation)
- Blood pressure (BP): assess orthostatic
- Weight

General Appearance

- Apparent state of health
- Appearance of comfort or distress
- Color/turgor of skin (check for dehydration caused by severe diarrhea)

Mouth and Throat
- Inspect for any mouth lesions (chronic diarrhea concern regarding IBD)

Eyes
- Inspect for any redness in eyes
- Inspect for exophthalmos and lid retraction

Neck
- Inspect for thyroid enlargement
- Palpate thyroid: size, consistency, contour, position, tenderness

Abdomen
- Inspect for contour, bruits, heaves, previous abdominal scars
- Auscultate for bowel sounds
- Palpate for masses, pain

Rectum
- Inspect for fissure, fistula
- Palpate for sphincter tone (fecal incontinence), visible or occult blood

CASE STUDY

History

Question	Response
How long have you had "loose stools"?	*3 days*
Is it getting better or worse or staying the same?	*The same*
How frequently have you had the "loose stools"	*Every 2 to 3 hours*
What does the stool look like?	*Semi-formed to liquid consistency, brown*
Do you have any associated symptoms? Fever? Abdominal pain? Nausea/vomiting?	*No fever, some abdominal cramping especially when having a bowel movement; some nausea, no vomiting*
Where do you live/reside? Facility?	*Live at home with husband and three children*
What is your occupation?	*Home day care provider*
Do you have any particular hobbies?	*No particular hobbies*
Have you traveled anywhere recently?	*No recent travel*
Have you traveled anywhere in the past year?	*Only to the mountains 2 hours away last summer*

Question	Response
What have you eaten in the past 24 hours, past 48 hours?	*I have been trying to eat bland foods. Yesterday I had a piece of pizza, which caused an increase in diarrhea and cramping.*
Have you regularly ingested any sugar-free foods (foods containing sorbitol)?	*No*
What recent medications are you taking?	*Only a women's multivitamin and vitamin D from Costco*

Physical Examination Findings

- VITAL SIGNS: temperature 99°F, respiratory rate (RR) 16, heart rate (HR) 90, BP 110/78, no orthostatic changes noted
- GENERAL APPEARANCE: well-developed female in no acute distress, appears slightly fatigued
- SKIN: good skin turgor noted, moist mucous membranes
- EYES: pupils equal, round, and reactive to light and accommodation (PERRLA), no injection, anicteric
- MOUTH: no oral lesions, teeth and gums in good repair
- NECK: no palpable lymph nodes noted, thyroid not enlarged
- ABDOMEN: positive bowel sounds (BS) in all four quadrants; no masses; no organomegaly noted; diffuse, mild, bilateral lower quadrant pain noted
- RECTUM: good sphincter tone; stool occult blood negative, no hemorrhoids, fissures noted

DIFFERENTIAL DIAGNOSIS

Differential Diagnosis	Viral	Bacterial	Protozoal
Duration of symptoms	< 2 to 3 days > 2 to 3 days	> 2 to 3 days	
Frequency	Every (q) 2 to 3 hours	Profuse	Variable
Fever	Low or none	High	Low or none
Abdominal pain, cramping	Mild	Severe	Moderate
Pus in stool	−	+	+ or −
Blood in stool	−	+	−
Previous antibiotics	−	+	−
Dehydration	Rare	More likely	Rare
Hours of overseas travel	Rare	More common	Common

DIAGNOSTIC EXAMS

Examination	Procedure Code	Cost	Results
Hemoccult Stool for occult blood	82270	$10 to $25	Testing for occult (hidden) blood is stool based. The best method for obtaining stool—digital examination of the rectum versus patient-submitted stool—is controversial. **Guiac based fecal occult blood test** • Test identifies hemoglobin by the presence of a peroxidate reaction, turns guiac-impregnated paper blue • A positive test is more likely with more blood in the GI tract • Dietary factors may influence the test results, though a restrictive diet may not be needed • High rate of false positives in healthy populations (80% of positive tests are felt to be false positives) • Positives in diarrhea need to look for causes of GI bleeding, such as infections in acute diarrhea, in chronic diarrhea concerns regarding IBD
Fecal leukocytes	89055	$35	The presence of leukocytes is an indicator of inflammation. Generally, the inflammation is a product of a bacteria–host interaction. Leukocytes are found in stools in the presence of infection with bacteria that invade the colonic mucosa (i.e., *Salmonella, Shigella, Yersinia,* and invasive *Escherichia coli*). Other disorders that may be associated with fecal leukocytes are ulcerative colitis and antibiotic-associated colitis. Fecal leukocytes are usually absent in diarrhea secondary to toxigenic bacteria, parasites, or virus. • Meta-analysis of diagnostic test accuracy estimates that for a peak sensitivity of 70% the specificity of fecal leukocytes was only 50% • There have been a number of studies showing variability of test performance • The presence of occult blood and fecal leukocytes supports a diagnosis of bacterial diarrhea in the context of the medical history and other diagnostic evaluations

Stool culture	87045	$70 to $294	• Stool cultures are useful in determining a bacterial cause for diarrhea. Low rate of positive stool cultures in most reports (2%–5%). Most episodes of diarrhea are self-limiting and the infection clears.
			• Useful after several days of supportive therapy if diarrhea does not resolve. Determining a bacterial cause is useful in patients with severe disease.
			• The following patients should have stool cultures on initial presentation:
			  a. Immunocompromised patients (HIV)
			  b. Patients with comorbidities that increase the risk for complications
			  c. Patients with more severe, inflammatory diarrhea
			  d. Patients with underlying IBD
			  e. Food handlers who may need negative cultures to return to work

(*continued*)

Examination	Procedure Code	Cost	Results

Stool for ova and parasites (O and P)	870177	$70 to $112	• Routine stool cultures identify *Salmonella, Camphylobacter,* and *Shigella*
			• Other organisms need to be specified, such as: *Clostridium difficile, Staphylococcus aureus*
			• Stool testing for O and P should be done if the patient is at risk for parasitic infection. Multiple stool samples should be collected at different times because shedding of parasites may be intermittent. Usually stool is collected at three different intervals or days.
			• Indications for O and P studies are:
			  a. Persistent diarrhea (acute to chronic)
			  b. Persistent diarrhea following travel to the developing world
			  c. Persistent diarrhea with exposure to infants in daycare centers
			  d. Diarrhea in men who have sex with men (MSM) or patients with AIDS
			  e. A community waterborne outbreak
			  f. Bloody diarrhea with few or no fecal leukocytes

CLINICAL DECISION MAKING

Case Study Analysis

The advanced practice nurse (APN) performs a detailed history and physical examination on the patient and finds the following data: diarrhea for the past 3 days with no fever, mild nausea, and no vomiting. Frequency is every 3 to 4 hours with liquid to soft light brown stools. Pertinent negatives include absence of fever, severe abdominal pain, vomiting, bloody stools, or weight loss. The patient has no chronic health problem and the only risk factor for a persistent diarrhea is that she is a home child care provider. The diagnosis at this time is viral gastroenteritis.

Diagnosis: Acute diarrhea of a viral etiology

DIZZINESS

Case Presentation: A previously healthy 47-year-old female presents to your clinic with a 4-day history of "dizziness."

INTRODUCTION TO COMPLAINT

- The complaint of dizziness is a common reason for patients 18 years and older to seek primary care clinic visits and accounts for an estimated 5% of primary care visits
- The vagueness of the complaint makes it challenging for clinicians to diagnose
- The complaint of dizziness involves a broad differential diagnosis, from the relatively simple to potentially serious conditions
- Ask open-ended questions about "dizziness" to classify it into one of four categories

Vertigo

- Illusory sensation of movement or spinning, usually arises from a disorder of the vestibular system
- Distinguish whether the vertigo is central (brainstem or cerebellar) or peripheral (vestibular) in origin
- Accounts for 45% to 54% of patients with dizziness
- Benign paroxysmal positional vertigo (BPPV), Ménière's disease, vestibular neuritis, and labyrinthitis are main causes of vertigo

Presyncope

- This sensation is associated with near-fainting or "nearly blacking out"
- Typically brief, lasting seconds or minutes, and is self-resolving
- Includes vasovagal attacks, orthostatic hypotension, or cardiac arrhythmias
- Many medications can cause presyncope

Disequilibrium

- This is a sense of imbalance, usually while walking
- Is a multifactorial disorder, commonly seen in elderly patients with impaired vision, peripheral neuropathy, decreased proprioception, and musculoskeletal problems causing gait instability, such as Parkinson's disease or multiple sclerosis
- Some disequilibrium can be exacerbated by medications, particularly in the elderly

Lightheadedness (Nonspecific Dizziness)

- This is a vague symptom characterized by disconnection with the environment
- Psychiatric disorders, such as depression, anxiety, and hyperventilation syndrome, can cause vague lightheadedness

HISTORY OF COMPLAINT

Symptomatology

Ask about the following characteristics of each symptom using open-ended questions:

- Onset (sudden or gradual)
- Chronology
- Improving or worsening
- Intermittent or constant
- Severity
- Timing (frequency, duration)
- Precipitating and aggravating factors
- Relieving factors
- Associated symptoms
- Effect on daily activities
- Previous diagnosis of similar episodes
- Previous treatment
- Efficacy of previous treatments

Directed Questions to Ask

- Was the onset sudden or gradual?
- Do you feel as though you or the room is spinning?
- Do you feel as though your balance is off?
- Do you feel like you are about to faint?
- Would you describe yourself as anxious or nervous?
- Do the episodes occur with any specific activity or movement?
- Do you have migraine headaches?
- Do you have nausea and vomiting?
- When do the episodes occur?
- How long do the episodes of dizziness last?
- Are there any neurologic deficits, such as extremity weakness or dysarthria?
- Do you have any hearing loss, tinnitus, or fullness in your ears?
- What medications are you taking?
- What other medical problems do you have?
- Are you now or have you recently been ill?
- Have you had any recent injury to your head or ear?
- Did you have dizziness before the head injury?
- Have you had any previous ear surgery?
- Is it associated with positional changes?
- Do you have any history of chronic middle ear infections?

Assessment: Cardinal Signs and Symptoms

In addition to the general characteristics outlined above, additional characteristics of specific symptoms should be elicited, as follows:

Head, Eyes, Ears, Nose, Throat (HEENT)
- Hearing loss
- Tinnitus
- Nystagmus (vertical, lateral, and/or rotary)
- Double vision or photophobia, diplopia

- Dysarthria
- Dysphagia

Respiratory
- Hypercapnia

Cardiovascular
- Palpitations
- Arrhythmias

Gastroenterology
- Nausea and vomiting

Psychiatric
- Stress

Neurology
- Ataxia
- Neurological focal deficits
- Headaches
- Paresthesia

Other Associated Symptoms
- Fever
- Malaise
- Diaphoresis
- Volume status

Medical History: General

- Medical conditions and surgeries
- Allergies
- Medication currently used (antihypertensive medications, ototoxic drugs, or psychotropic drugs)
- Recent viral and bacterial respiratory infections
- Family history of stroke, transient ischemic attacks (TIA), multiple sclerosis, cardiac disease, diabetes mellitus, or hypertension
- Social history of smoking

Medical History: Specific to Complaint

- Trauma to head, ear, or neck, such as whiplash
- History of ear surgeries or ear infections
- Migraine headache

PHYSICAL EXAMINATION

Vital Signs

- Temperature
- Pulse
- Respiration
- SpO_2 (oxygen saturation)
- Blood pressure (BP)
- Orthostatic BP (systolic blood pressure [SBP] increase of 20 mmHg, diastolic blood pressure [DBP] decrease of 10 mmHg, heart rate (HR) increase of 30)

General Appearance

- Apparent state of health
- Appearance of distress
- Color
- Difficulty with gait or balance
- Volume status

HEENT

- HEAD: any trauma, tenderness to palpation
- EYES: conjunctiva and sclera, fundi, extraocular muscles (EOM)
- EARS: outer and middle ear canal

Respiratory

- Respiratory rate
- Auscultation

Cardiovascular

- Auscultation
- Jugular venous distension (JVD)
- Extremities for edema

Gastroenterology

- Bowel tones
- Tenderness
- Mass or enlarged organs

Neurology

- Dix-Hallpike maneuver
- Cranial nerves
- Mental status
- Motor system
- Sensory system
- Reflexes
- Romberg test
- Ataxia

Associated Systems for Assessment

A complete assessment should include the skin and lymph system.

CASE STUDY

History

Question	Response
Was the onset sudden or gradual?	*It came on suddenly*
Do you feel as though you or the room is spinning or do you feel light headed?	*I feel like the room is spinning*
Do you feel as though your balance is off as you have difficulty walking?	*I do feel like my balance is off since the room is spinning*
Do you feel like you are about to faint?	*No, I do not feel like I am going to faint*
Would you describe yourself as anxious or nervous?	*No, I am not anxious or nervous*

Question	Response
What makes it worse?	*Moving around makes it worse*
What makes it better?	*Not moving and staying in a flat position on the bed*
Do you have any fever, chills, weight loss, or night sweats?	*No*
Do the episodes occur with any specific activity or movement?	*When I move or stand up, it makes it worse*
Do you have migraine headaches?	*No, I do not have a history of migraine*
Do you have nausea and vomiting?	*I feel nauseous but no vomiting*
How long do the episodes of dizziness last?	*Sometimes minutes but sometimes longer when I am moving around*
Are there any neurologic deficits, such as extremity weakness or dysarthria?	*No, I do not have any neurological deficits*
Do you have any hearing loss, tinnitus, or fullness in your ears?	*No, I have no ear complaints*
What medications are you taking?	*I am not taking any medications currently*
What other medical problems do you have?	*I am otherwise healthy*
Are you now or have you recently been ill?	*No, I have not been ill recently*
Have you had any recent injury to your head, ear, or neck, such as whiplash? If so, did you have dizziness before the head injury?	*No, I had no injury recently*
Have you had any previous ear surgery?	*No, I do not have any history of ear surgery*
Have you ever had these symptoms previously?	*No, I never had these symptoms in the past*

Physical Examination Findings

- VITAL SIGNS: BP 110/75; heart rate (HR) 65 bpm and regular; respiratory rate (RR) 14 breaths/min; temperature 99.3°F
- GENERAL APPEARANCE: well developed, well nourished (WDWN), sitting comfortably on the examination table
- SKIN: no rash; nails without cyanosis or clubbing
- HEENT: normocephalic, atraumatic, pupils equal, round, and reactive to light and accommodation (PERRLA), constrict from 5 mm to 2 mm, disc margins are sharp, fundi without hemorrhages or exudates; external ear canals patent; tympanic membranes with good cone of light; sinus nontender; oral mucosa pink, without enlarged tonsils; dentition good; pharynx has mild erythema, but there are no exudates
- NECK: supple, without thyromegaly; no cervical lymphadenopathy
- THORAX AND LUNGS: thorax symmetric, with good expansion, lungs resonant; breath sounds vesicular

- CARDIOVASCULAR: regular rate and rhythm (RRR), jugular venous pressure (JVP) 6 cm above right atrium; carotid upstrokes brisk, without bruits; no murmurs, rubs, and gallops (MRG), normal S1, S2; no S3, S4
- ABDOMEN: bowel sounds active; soft and nontender, no hepatosplenomegaly (HSM)
- PERIPHERAL VASCULAR/EXTREMITIES: extremities without edema; pedal pulses are 2+ bilaterally
- MUSCULOSKELETAL (MSK): full range of motion (ROM) in all joints, no swelling or deformities
- NEUROLOGIC: mental status—patient is oriented to person, place, and time
    - Cranial nerves (CN): CN II through XII intact including EOM
    - Motor: good bulk and tone; strength is 5/5 throughout
    - Cerebellar: nystagmus with leftward gaze, rapid alternating movements (RAMs) finger to nose and heel to shin are intact; gait with normal base; negative pronator drift; negative Romberg test
    - Sensory: pinprick and light touch are intact and symmetric throughout
    - Reflexes: 2+ and symmetric
    - Dix-Hallpike maneuver: elicited rotational nystagmus in the left eye

DIFFERENTIAL DIAGNOSIS

Differential Diagnosis	Benign Paroxysmal Positional Vertigo	Ménière's Disease	Vestibular Neuritis
Onset	Sudden	Sudden	Sudden
Provoking factors	Head change movements	None	None
Episodic or recurrent	Recurrent	Recurrent	Single episodes
Duration of episodes	Seconds to minutes	Last several minutes to hours but no longer than 24 hours	Days to weeks
Tinnitus	Not common	Unilateral or bilateral tinnitus	Not affected
Nausea/vomiting	Often associated with nausea	Often	Usually
Hearing loss	Not affected	Fluctuating, positive unilateral, or bilateral hearing loss	Not affected
Nystagmus	Rotatory	Horizontal; lessens with focus on gaze	Horizontal; lessens or disappears with focus on gaze
Headache	Not common	Increased	Not common
Weakness	Rarely	Rarely	Sometimes
Gait instability	Unilateral instability	Walking preserved	Walking preserved

(*continued*)

Differential Diagnosis	Benign Paroxysmal Positional Vertigo	Ménière's Disease	Vestibular Neuritis
Associated neurologic symptoms	None	None	Falls toward side of lesion, no brainstem symptoms
Photophobia	Sometimes	Sometimes	Not common
Vertigo	Spinning dizziness, rotational component	Rotational vertigo, severe and incapacitating at times	Vertigo present
Presyncope/ syncope	Not common	Not common	Not common
Vomiting	Uncommon but possible	May be associated with vomiting	May be associated with vomiting
Phonophobia	Not common	Common	Not common
Fullness in ears	Rarely	Unilateral or bilateral	Not common

DIAGNOSTIC EXAMINATION

Examination	Procedure Code	Cost	Indications and Interpretation
CT without contrast	70450	$1290	• Superior to MRI in detection of hemorrhage within the first 24 to 48 hours • Evaluation of sinus disease and temporal bone disease • Overall is a less sensitive test than MRI for early infarcts and small mass lesions
MRI (magnetic resonance angiography [MRA]) stroke protocol	70551– 70553	$4097	• MRI is superior to CT for the diagnosis of vertigo because of its superior ability to visualize the posterior fossa • Order to determine cause of vertigo or acoustic neuroma • New headache accompanying vertigo • Evaluation of essentially all intracranial diseases except those listed above for CT
BMP (basic metabolic panel)	80048	$119	• Glucose: Energy • BUN (blood urea nitrogen): Waste produced is filtered out of the blood by the kidneys; conditions that affect the kidney have the potential to affect the amount of urea in the blood (dehydration) • Creatinine: Waste product produced in the muscles is filtered out of the blood by the kidneys, so blood levels are a good indication of how well the kidneys are working

(continued)

Examination	Procedure Code	Cost	Indications and Interpretation
EKG	93000	$150	• Heart valve abnormalities • Global and regional left ventricular function (normal contraction) • Estimate of the ejection fraction or amount of blood pumped out by each ventricular contraction • Identify a mural thrombosis (blood clot in the ventricle wall)
CBC (complete blood count)	85025	$75	• White blood count (WBC) • High WBC can indicate an infection (or stress) • Hemoglobin (Hgb) and hematocrit (Hct) • Anemia can be seen due to nutritional deficiencies, blood loss, destruction of blood cells internally, or failure to produce blood in the bone marrow

Examination	Procedure Code	Cost
TSH (thyroid stimulating hormone)	84439	$39
Free T4 (thyroxine)	84439	$70
T3 (triiodothyronine)	84479	$79

TSH	Serum Free T4	Serum T3	Assessment
Normal	Normal	Normal	Euthyroid
High	Low	Normal or low	Primary hypothyroidism
High	Normal	Normal	Subclinical hypothyroidism
Low	High or normal	High	Hyperthyroidism
Low	Normal	Normal	Subclinical hyperthyroidism

CLINICAL DECISION MAKING

Case Study Analysis

The clinician performs the assessment and physical examination on the patient and finds the following data: sudden onset of vertigo, especially with positional changes, with nausea and vomiting with no neurological deficits. Noted positive Dix-Hallpike maneuver that initiated rotational nystagmus on the left side.

Diagnosis: *Benign paroxysmal positional vertigo*

- BPPV is the most common form of vertigo, accounting for nearly 50% of patients with peripheral vestibular dysfunction
- BPPV is caused by calcium debris in the semicircular canals (canalithiasis)

Generally, medications are not recommended for the treatment of the brief episodes of vertigo associated with BPPV. However, the following vestibular suppressant medications can be used as premedication with liberatory maneuvers in patients with acute vertigo with nausea and emesis.

Clinical Pearl
- Although most patients with dizziness do not need to be referred to a subspecialist, clinicians should consider referral to the appropriate subspecialist (e.g., otolaryngologist or neurologist) if the diagnosis is not clear.

EAR DISCHARGE

Case Presentation: *A 57-year-old man presents to your clinic with a complaint of left ear drainage.*

INTRODUCTION TO COMPLAINT

Ear discharge can be caused by several conditions, including rupture of the tympanic membrane, infection or trauma of the external ear, or as a result of cerumen that has softened (i.e., due to increased temperature).

Bacterial Infections

Ear discharge can be related to a bacterial infection that has caused increased fluid accumulation and inflammation behind the tympanic membrane leading to rupture. Bacterial infections in the ear canal or external ear may have exudate present that drains from the ear.

Allergic Conditions

Allergic conditions (e.g., seasonal and environmental factors) or allergies to a specific irritant (e.g., animal dander) can cause inflammation in the upper respiratory tract, including the Eustachian tubes. This can cause fluid accumulation in the absence of bacterial infection. Although an infection may not be present, the pressure from the fluid accumulation can still cause pressure inside the middle ear. With excessive increase in pressure, the tympanic membrane can rupture, leading to drainage from the ear.

Trauma

Ear discharge can be caused by direct trauma to the ear. The drainage may be bloody and directly related to the trauma, or the trauma may lead to a point of entry for an infectious agent, resulting in drainage that is more exudative in appearance.

HISTORY OF COMPLAINT

Symptomatology

Ask about the following characteristics of each symptom using open-ended questions:

- Onset
- Contributing factors: history prior to drainage
- Exposure to illness
- Exposure to second- or third-hand smoke
- Associated symptoms

- Description of drainage
- Aggravating factors
- Alleviating factors
- Effect on hearing
- History of similar episodes
- Previous treatments tried

Directed Questions to Ask

- Was the onset sudden or gradual?
- Have you had any ear pain?
- Have you had sinus or nasal congestion?
- Have you had a sore throat?
- What does the ear drainage look like?
- Is the drainage from just one ear, or both?
- Have you been exposed to anyone who is sick?
- Do you or anyone in your household smoke?
- Has your hearing changed?
- Have you had a fever?
- Have you been coughing?
- Have you been short of breath?
- Has your appetite changed?
- Have you vomited?
- Have you ever had anything like this before?
- If yes, what treatment did you receive?

Assessment: Cardinal Signs and Symptoms

In addition to the directed questions listed above, the following need to be included in the assessment:

Ears
- Drainage: color, consistency, odor, amount
- Edema
- Erythema
- Hearing change

Eyes
- Conjunctivitis
- Vision change
- Pain

Nose
- Congestion

Mouth and Throat
- Sore throat
- Cough
- Dental status
- Dysphagia
- Oral lesions

Neck
- Pain
- Decreased range of motion (ROM)
- Swelling
- Enlarged glands

Nervous System
- Dermatome involvement

Skin
- Rash

Other Associated Symptoms
- Fever
- Fatigue
- Headache

Medical History: General
- Medical conditions and surgeries
- Allergies (seasonal or other)
- Current medications

Medical History: Specific to Complaint
- Frequent ear infections
- Smoking history
- History of ear surgery
- Trauma to ear
- Recent history of swimming
- Recent history of travel

PHYSICAL EXAMINATION
Vital Signs
- Temperature
- Pulse
- Respiration
- SpO_2 (oxygen saturation)
- Blood pressure

General Appearance
- Apparent state of health
- Current level of comfort or distress
- Skin color and temperature
- Nutritional status
- Hydration status
- Hygiene
- Appearance in accordance with stated age
- Gait or balance difficulty

Ear Inspection
- EXTERNAL EAR: color, structure, swelling, presence of cerumen
- CANAL: redness, swelling; presence, character, and amount of exudate
- TYMPANIC MEMBRANE: intact, color, light reflex, landmarks, presence of effusion, injection, apparent pressure

Eye Inspection
- Drainage
- Color

Nose Inspection
- Congestion
- Drainage
- Pallor

Mouth and Throat Inspection
- Color
- Presence of lesions
- Symmetry
- Exudate

Neck Inspection and Palpation
- Symmetry
- Swelling
- Masses
- Active ROM
- Thyroid: size, symmetry, masses

Neurologic Examination
- Facial nerve assessment
- Hearing test

Associated Systems for Assessment
A complete assessment should include the respiratory system, abdominal assessment, general skin inspection, and general extremities assessment.

CASE STUDY
History

Question	Response
Was the onset sudden or gradual?	*It came on gradually*
Have you had any ear pain?	*Yes, but it has gotten a little better*
What does the drainage look like?	*Clear with some wax in it*
Have you been exposed to anyone who is sick?	*Not that I know of*
Do you or anyone in your household smoke?	*No*

Question	Response
Is the pain just in the ear, or is there pain in other areas?	*A little in my throat, but mostly my ear*
Are you able to describe the pain?	*It's a sharp ache*
Is the pain interfering with activities?	*Some, it's hard to focus*
Have you noticed a hearing change?	*My left ear feels muffled*
Does anything make the pain better?	*Not that I've noticed*
Does anything make the pain worse?	*When I take a shower*
Have you had a fever?	*No*
Have you had a runny nose?	*Yes*
Have you been coughing?	*Occasionally I have a dry cough*
Have you been short of breath?	*No*
Has your appetite changed?	*No*
Have you vomited?	*No*
Have you ever had anything like this before?	*No, I've had ear aches before, but not drainage*
If yes, what treatment did you receive?	*Antibiotics and allergy pills*
Have you ever had the chicken pox, cold sores, or shingles?	*No*

Physical Examination Findings

- VITAL SIGNS: 98.9°F; respiratory rate (RR) 14; heart rate (HR) 76; blood pressure (BP) 126/84
- GENERAL APPEARANCE: well-developed, healthy appearing male
- EAR INSPECTION: right ear—external ear normal, canal without erythema or exudate, small amount of cerumen, tympanic membrane pearly grey, intact with light reflex and bony landmarks present; left ear—external ear normal, canal with white exudate and crusting, no visualization of tympanic membrane or bony landmarks, no light reflex
- EYE INSPECTION: bilateral mild conjunctivitis, anicteric, pupils equal, round, and reactive to light and accommodation (PERRLA), extraocular movements intact
- NOSE INSPECTION: nares are patent with soft tissue edema, pale, with moderate clear rhinorrhea
- MOUTH AND THROAT INSPECTION: no oral lesions, teeth and gums in good repair, oropharynx moderately erythematous with postnasal drip
- NECK INSPECTION AND PALPATION: no cervical lymphadenopathy, soft, supple, fully active ROM, thyroid normal size without mass
- NEUROLOGIC EXAMINATION: hearing grossly normal, sensation of face normal and symmetric, gait normal

- CHEST: lungs are clear in all fields, heart rate and rhythm are regular without murmur or rub
- ABDOMEN: soft, nontender without mass or organomegaly
- SKIN: no rashes
- EXTREMITIES: no joint pain or swelling

DIFFERENTIAL DIAGNOSIS

Differential Diagnosis	Bacterial	Allergic	Trauma
Onset	Abrupt	Gradual	Abrupt
Fever	+ or −	−	−
Chills	+ or −	−	−
Ear pain	Common	Common	Common
Sore throat	+ or −	+ or −	−
Nasal congestion	+ or −	+	−
Nasal discharge	+ or −	+	−
Postnasal drip	−	+	−
Cough	+ or −	+	−
Fatigue	+ or −	+ or −	−
Headache	+ or −	+ or −	+ or −
Nodes in neck	+ or −	+ or −	−

DIAGNOSTIC EXAMINATION

Examination	Procedure Code	Cost	Results
Otoscopy	NA	Included in office visit	Visualization of the ear canal and tympanic membrane to assess for presence of foreign body, signs of trauma, erythema, effusion, or rupture

CLINICAL DECISION MAKING

Case Study Analysis

The advanced practice nurse performs the assessment and physical examination on the patient and finds the following positives: gradual onset of left ear pain with eventual rupture and drainage of effusion, nasal congestion, mild sore throat with postnasal drip, and occasional dry cough. Pertinent negatives include lack of trauma to ear, no recent swimming, and lack of fever or loss of hearing.

> *Diagnosis:* Otitis media with effusion and rupture

EAR PAIN

Case Presentation: A 3-year-old girl presents to your clinic with a complaint of left ear pain for 2 days. She arrives in the company of her mother.

INTRODUCTION TO COMPLAINT

Ear pain can range from mildly uncomfortable to very painful. It can resolve spontaneously or progress to more serious infections involving the surrounding tissue, even, though rare, the brain. Several conditions can cause ear pain.

Viral or Bacterial Infections

Often ear pain can be related to an infection that has caused increased fluid and inflammation behind the tympanic membrane. Bacterial infections may also occur in the ear canal or external ear, causing inflammation and/or cellulitis of the soft tissue.

Allergic Conditions

Allergic conditions, such as seasonal and environmental conditions, or allergies to a specific irritant (i.e., animal dander) can cause inflammation in the upper respiratory tract, including the Eustachian tubes. This can cause fluid accumulation in the absence of bacterial infection. Although an infection may not be present, the pressure from the fluid accumulation can still cause pressure inside the middle ear, thereby causing sensation of pain.

Neuropathic Conditions

Sometimes pain that is caused by nerve root irritation can present as ear pain. This can be caused by impingement of a nerve (auricular or temporal nerves), or may be related to activation of a viral infection, such as herpes simplex virus (HSV) or herpes zoster.

Trauma/Foreign Body

Ear pain can be caused by direct trauma to the ear or by the presence of a foreign body (FB). This is typically due to a specific event.

Referred Pain

Pain felt in the ear may have a point of origin that is in the surrounding anatomic structures and is referred and/or radiating to the ear. The site of origin may be the sinus cavities, the throat, the eye, the thyroid, cervical spine, or surrounding support muscles.

HISTORY OF COMPLAINT
Symptomatology

Ask about the following characteristics of each symptom using open-ended questions:

- Onset
- Exposure to illness
- Exposure to second-hand or third-hand smoke
- History of health conditions, specifically exposure to herpes simplex virus (HSV) or herpes zoster
- Location of pain
- Radiation
- Character of the pain
- Aggravating factors
- Alleviating factors
- Associated symptoms
- Effect on activity level
- Effect on hearing
- History of similar episodes
- Previous treatments tried

Directed Questions to Ask

- Was the onset sudden or gradual?
- Has she been exposed to anyone who is sick?
- Does she or anyone in your household smoke?
- Is the pain just in the ear, or is there pain in other areas?
- How does she describe the pain?
- Is the pain interfering with activities?
- Has her hearing changed?
- Does anything make the pain better?
- Does anything make the pain worse?
- Has she had a fever?
- Has she had a runny nose?
- Has she been coughing?
- Has she been short of breath?
- Has her appetite changed?
- Has she vomited?
- Has she ever had anything like this before?
- If yes, what treatment did she receive?
- Has she ever had the chicken pox, cold sores, or shingles?

Assessment: Cardinal Signs and Symptoms

In addition to the directed questions listed above, the following need to be included in the assessment:

Ears
- Drainage
- Edema
- Erythema
- Hearing change

Eyes
- Conjunctivitis
- Vision change
- Pain

Nose
- Congestion

Mouth and Throat
- Sore throat
- Cough
- Dental status
- Dysphagia
- Oral lesions

Neck
- Pain
- Decreased range of motion (ROM)
- Swelling
- Enlarged glands

Nervous System
- Dermatome involvement

Skin
- Rash

Other Associated Symptoms
- Fever
- Fatigue
- Headache

Medical History: General
- Medial conditions and surgeries
- Allergies (seasonal or other)
- Current medications

Medical History: Specific to Complaint
- Frequent ear infections
- Smoking history
- History of ear surgery
- Trauma to ear
- Recent history of swimming
- Recent history of travel

PHYSICAL EXAMINATION
Vital Signs
- Temperature
- Pulse
- Respiration
- SpO_2 (oxygen saturation)
- Blood pressure

General Appearance

- Apparent state of health
- Current level of comfort or distress
- Skin color and temperature
- Nutritional status
- Hydration status
- Hygiene
- Appearance in accordance with stated age
- Gait or balance difficulty

Ear Inspection

- External ear: color, structure, swelling, presence of cerumen
- Canal: redness, swelling, presence of exudate
- Tympanic membrane (TM): intact, color, light reflex, landmarks, presence of effusion, injection, apparent pressure

Eye Inspection

- Drainage
- Color

Nose Inspection

- Congestion
- Drainage
- Pallor

Mouth and Throat Inspection

- Color
- Presence of lesions
- Symmetry
- Exudate

Neck Inspection and Palpation

- Symmetry
- Swelling
- Masses
- Active ROM
- Thyroid: size, symmetry, masses

Neurologic Examination

- Facial nerve assessment
- Hearing test

Associated Systems for Assessment

A complete assessment should include the respiratory system, abdominal assessment, general skin inspection, and general extremities assessment.

CASE STUDY
History

Question	Response
Was the onset sudden or gradual?	*It was sudden*
Has the child been exposed to anyone who is sick?	*She goes to day care, so it's hard to tell*
Do you or anyone in your household smoke?	*No*
Is the pain just in the ear, or is there pain in other areas?	*It just seems to be the ear*
Is she able to describe the pain?	*No*
Is the pain interfering with activities?	*No*
Have you noticed a hearing change?	*No*
Does anything make the pain better?	*No*
Does anything make the pain worse?	*No*
Has she had a fever?	*No*
Has she had a runny nose?	*She did about a week ago, but it's getting better*
Has she been coughing?	*Occasionally*
Has she been short of breath?	*No*
Has her appetite changed?	*No*
Has she vomited?	*No*
Has she ever had anything like this before?	*Yes, the same time last year*
If yes, what treatment did she receive?	*Antibiotics*
Has she ever had chicken pox, cold sores, or shingles?	*No*

Physical Examination Findings

- VITAL SIGNS: 98.5°F, respiratory rate (RR) 22, heart rate (HR) 110, blood pressure (BP) 92/60
- GENERAL APPEARANCE: well-developed, healthy-appearing child; fussy, but active
- EAR INSPECTION: right ear—external ear normal, canal without erythema or exudate, small amount of cerumen, tympanic membrane (TM) pearly grey, intact with light reflex and bony landmarks present; left ear—external ear normal, canal without erythema or exudate, small amount of cerumen, TM erythematous and bulging
- EYE INSPECTION: no injection; anicteric; pupils equal, round, and reactive to light and accommodation (PERRLA); extraocular movements intact
- NOSE INSPECTION: nares are patent, no edema, minimal clear rhinorrhea
- MOUTH AND THROAT INSPECTION: no oral lesions, teeth and gums in good repair

- NECK INSPECTION AND PALPATION: no cervical lymphadenopathy, soft, supple, fully active ROM, thyroid normal size without mass
- NEUROLOGIC EXAMINATION: hearing grossly normal, sensation of face normal and symmetric, gait normal
- CHEST: lungs are clear in all fields, heart rate and rhythm are regular without murmur or rub
- ABDOMEN: soft, nontender without mass or organomegaly
- SKIN: no rashes
- EXTREMITIES: no joint pain or swelling

DIFFERENTIAL DIAGNOSIS

Differential Diagnosis	Bacterial	Allergic	Neuropathic	Trauma/FB	Referred
Onset	Abrupt	Gradual	Either	Abrupt	Either
Fever	+ or −	−	−	−	+ or −
Chills	+ or −	−	−	−	+ or −
Sore throat	+ or −	+ or −	−	−	+ or −
Nasal congestion	+ or −	+	-	−	+ or −
Nasal discharge	+ or −	+	−	−	+ or −
Postnasal drip	−	+	−	−	−
Cough	+ or −	+	−	−	+ or −
Fatigue	+ or −	+ or −	+ or −	−	+ or −
Headache	+ or −	+ or −	+ or −	+ or -	+ or −
Nodes in neck	+ or −	+ or −	+ or −	−	+ or −
Thyroid disease	−	−	−	−	+ or −
History of neck injury	−	−	+ or −	+ or −	+ or −
Muscle spasm	−	−	+ or −	+ or −	+ or −
History of HSV	−	−	+ or −	−	+ or −
Dermatome Involvement	−	−	+	−	+ or −
History of temporomandibular joint disorders (TMJ)	−	−	−	−	+

DIAGNOSTIC EXAMINATION

Examination	Procedure Code	Cost	Results
Otoscopy	NA	Included in office visit	Visualization of the ear canal and TM to assess for presence of FB, signs of trauma, erythema, effusion, or rupture
Tympanometry	92567	$41	The measurement of pressure behind the TM does not determine whether or not an infectious process is present. Normal pressure levels are between −150 and +25 daPa. An elevated pressure indicates increased pressure behind the TM. Further assessment is necessary to determine the cause of increased pressure.
Herpes simplex immunoglobulin G (IgG)	86694 86695 86696	$13 to $17	If ear pain is neuropathic in nature with presence or history of oral lesions, this test would help determine whether nerve root irritation is a causative factor If this test returns a positive result in the presence of additional examination findings consistent with neuropathic pain, antiviral therapy may be considered to assist with suppression of HSV. Additionally, use of steroidal agents may assist with pain reduction.

CLINICAL DECISION MAKING

Case Study Analysis

The nurse practitioner performs the assessment and physical examination on the child and finds the following pertinent positives: day care–attending child with sudden onset of left ear pain without radiation to other areas and without discharge, with a history of similar occurrence last year. Left TM injected with effusion. Pertinent negative is absence of fever.

> *Diagnosis:* Acute otitis media (left ear)

ELBOW PAIN

Case Presentation: A 37-year-old male states, "My right elbow has been hurting for weeks."

INTRODUCTION TO COMPLAINT

Elbow pain results from one of the following:

- Repetitive or overuse syndromes
- Tendon and muscle pain due to work or sports activities
- Inflammation
- Joint capsule inflammation of the internal capsule due to arthritis, gout, or infection
- Swelling
- Bursitis or swelling of the olecranon bursa from direct pressure or trauma
- Trauma
- Bone pain due to fracture of the bone due to trauma or severe stress
- Nerve entrapment
- Nerve pain or numbness and tingling along the median or ulnar nerve due to compression
- Tendonitis

HISTORY OF COMPLAINT

Symptomatology

Ask about the following characteristics of each symptom using open-ended questions:

- Onset: Gradual or abrupt
- Timing and duration: Intermittent or constant
- Intensity: Severity of pain on a scale of 0 to 10
- Character: Is the pain sharp, dull, aching, burning?
- Radiation: Does the pain radiate into the shoulder, forearm, or wrist?
- Triggering: What movements trigger the pain?
- Alleviating: What lessens or resolves the pain?
- Effect on daily activity or sport
- Previous injury or treatment

Directed Questions to Ask

- Can you describe the injury from beginning to end? (if there was an acute injury)
- Was there immediate pain or swelling or did that occur later?

- Specifically where does the elbow hurt, can you put a finger on it?
- What types of movement makes the pain worse?
- Does the joint ever lock?
- Do you have weakness of your handgrip or difficulty lifting?
- Has anyone pulled on your elbow?
- Do you play a particular sport or have a hobby that uses your arms, elbows, wrist, or hand?
- Do you have any numbness or tingling?
- Do you have pain that wakes you up at night?
- Do you have any other joint pains? Have there been previous injuries?

Assessment: Cardinal Signs and Symptoms

- Pain over lateral elbow
- Pain over medial elbow
- Swelling over elbow
- Decreased range of motion

Medical History: General

- Medical history of gout, osteoarthritis, or rheumatoid arthritis
- Family history of gout, osteoarthritis, or rheumatoid arthritis
- Medications
- Allergies to medications
- Social history, including occupation, habits, and activities

Medical History: Specific to Complaint

- Medical history of gout, osteoarthritis, or rheumatoid arthritis
- Family history of gout, osteoarthritis, or rheumatoid arthritis

PHYSICAL EXAMINATION

- Vital signs
- General appearance

Objective

Physical examination of the elbow or any joint requires a review of basic anatomy of the joint.

Anatomy
- Humerus: The medial and lateral epicondyles form prominent bony landmarks of the distal humerus.
- Ulna: The proximal ulna articulates with the humerus. The olecranon process or point of the posterior elbow joint is part of the ulna.
- Radius: The proximal radial head articulates with the lateral elbow joint and allows for pronation and supination of the forearm.
- Olecranon bursa: This is an external bursa that lies over the olecranon or point of the elbow joint.

Neuromuscular
- Triceps extends the forearm (C7)
- The biceps flexes the forearm (C5 and C6)
- The brachioradialis assists with pronation (C6)
- The extensor carpi radialis longus extends and abducts the hand and wrists (C6)

- The supinator turns palms forward or supinates the forearm (C6 and C7)
- Ulnar and collateral ligaments stabilize the elbow joint

Neurological Anatomy
There are three nerves that innervate the elbow joint:

- Ulnar: medial side attaches to flexors
- Median: attached to pronators and passes through the carpal tunnel at the wrist
- Radial: provides sensation to the posterior forearm and moves extensor muscles
- Cervical nerves C5 and C6 may cause radicular pain and numbness in the elbow joint

Range of Motion of the Elbow
Flexion, extension, supination, and pronation

Musculoskeletal examinations should be performed in a systemic manner and include the following:

- Inspection and palpation
- Range of motion
- Strength testing of muscles above and below the joint
- Special test
- Reflexes and nerve testing
- Vascular status

Inspection and Palpation
- Starting with the anterior elbow in supination, observe and palpate the antecubital fossa for tenderness or masses.
- The biceps tendon and muscle is located superior to the fossa and a biceps tendon rupture would cause a palpable mass above the fossa.
- Observe and palpate the olecranon or the posterior elbow for tenderness or swelling.
- Bursitis is a common cause of nontraumatic swelling here and may be tender or nontender.
- Inspect and palpate the lateral elbow for tenderness, which may indicate "tennis elbow."
- If there has been trauma, tenderness over the radial head may indicate a fracture.
- Inspect and palpate the medial elbow for tenderness, which may indicate "golfers elbow."
- If there has been trauma to the elbow, there may be tenderness along the ulnar collateral ligament.
- Asses the ulnar nerve by tapping or performing Tinel's sign posterior to the medial epicondyle.
- If painful, this may indicate ulnar nerve injury.

Range of Motion
- Flexion/extension: 0 to 145 degrees
- Pronation: 80 to 90 degrees
- Supination: 85 to 90 degrees

Strength Testing
Test muscles against resistance on scale of 0 to 5 for:

- Flexion
- Extension
- Pronation
- Supination

Test Ligaments Against Resistance

Exert pressure on the medial (varus) side then laterally (valgus side) and feel for an opening on the opposite side indicating a torn or weakened ligament.

Reflexes

- Biceps (C5)
- Triceps (C7)

Tinel's Sign

Evaluate the ulnar nerve by tapping above the medial epicondyle. If there is tingling, this may mean there is ulnar nerve entrapment or cubital tunnel syndrome.

Vascular Status

Brachial and radial pulse should document that there is a normal vascular supply, especially if there has been an acute injury.

CASE STUDY

History

The patient is a 37-year-old male who is usually healthy but has a nagging pain in the right elbow for the past 2 weeks. He has tried taking ibuprofen and icing it, but it does not feel better. The pain is constant but worse when he picks up a heavy suitcase. He plays tennis 2 hours three times a week, but a month ago he increased to 2 hours a day. He does not have any other joint pain, stiffness, fever, or fatigue.

Question	Response
Did the pain start suddenly or gradually?	*Kinda gradual*
Was there any trauma or injury?	*No*
Is there any stiffness, heat, or swelling?	*No*
Is it stiff or hard to move?	*No, I can do everything with it*
Do you have any tingling or numbness?	*No*
Have you changed your routine activities?	*Yes, I am playing tennis daily now*
Have you ever injured the joint before?	*No, I'm pretty lucky*
Do any other joints hurt?	*No, just the right elbow*
Is there a family history of arthritis	*No, just heart disease in my dad*

Physical Examination Findings

- GENERAL APPEARANCE: athletic male in no acute distress
- NECK: full range of motion, nontender C spine
- SHOULDER: no deformity, nontender, full range of motion
- LEFT ELBOW: no deformity, nontender, full range of motion
- RIGHT ELBOW: no deformity, tender over the lateral epicondyle, pain with extension of wrist against resistance, no pain with supination or pronation
- TINEL'S SIGN: negative

- STRENGTH: biceps, triceps, supination, and pronation 5/5; valgus and varus ligaments intact
- VASCULAR: brachial and radial pulse 2+ and equal
- NEUROLOGY: sensation intact to C6, C7, C8 light touch and sharp; brachial and bracho-radialis (BR) reflex 2+ and equal

Most common causes of elbow pain are:

Lateral Epicondylitis	Medial Epicondylitis
History of playing tennis or racquet sport	History of golfing, or flexing the wrist
Pain over the lateral aspect of the elbow	Pain over the medial aspect of the elbow
Pain worse on lifting heavy objects	Pain worse on lifting heavy objects
Physical examination	Physical examination
Tender over the lateral epicondyle	Tender over the medial epicondyle
Pain worse on extending the wrist against resistance	Pain worse on flexing the wrist against resistance
No pain with full range of motion	No pain with full range of motion

DIFFERENTIAL DIAGNOSIS

Differential Diagnosis	Epicondylitis	Fracture	Gout	Arthritis
Pain	Yes, lateral or medial	Yes, diffuse over joint	Yes, red, warm, diffuse pain	Yes, over joint lines
Range of motion	Decreased	Decreased	Decreased	Decreased
Edema	No	Yes	Yes	Slight
Decreased strength	Mild, due to pain	Yes	Due to pain	Due to pain
Numbness	No	Possible	No	No

DIAGNOSTIC EXAMINATION

Examination	Procedure Code	Cost	Indication/Interpretation
X-ray, plain film	733120	$200	Trauma, weakness, locking; may reveal calcification or fracture
MRI	74200	$850	Suspected tendon rupture or soft tissues pathology

CLINICAL DECISION MAKING

Case Study Analysis

The clinician performs a history and physical examination and finds the following data:

- The pertinent positives are history of pain in the lateral elbow after increasing the number of hours the patient plays tennis.
- The pain is worse when the patient lifts heavy objects, and is partially relieved with rest.
- There is no numbness, tingling, or weakness to suggest nerve involvement.
- The physical examination confirms tenderness over the lateral epicondyle with normal joint motion otherwise.
- In the presence of full range of motion without pain, arthritis or gout are less likely.

Diagnosis: Lateral epicondylitis. Lateral epicondylitis is the most common cause of tendonitis. It is a clinical diagnosis and rarely is any diagnostic study needed unless there is a history of injury or weakness or nerve deficits are noted on examination.

Clinical Pearl
- Painless swelling of the olecranon process is common. It is external to the joint and appears as a fluid-filled sac. This is olecranon bursitis. If it is associated with increased warmth and redness or pain, aspiration of the fluid must be done to rule out infection.

FURTHER READING

Chumbley, E. M., O'Connor, F. G., & Nirschl, R. P. (2000). Evaluation of overuse elbow injuries. *American Family Physician, 61*(3), 691–700.

Ferri, F. F. (2011). *Ferri's clinical advisor.* St. Louis, MO: Mosby.

Miller, M. D., Hart, J. A., & MacKnight, J. M. (2010). *Essential orthopaedics.* Philadelphia, PA: Saunders.

ENLARGED LYMPH NODES

Case Presentation: *A 64-year-old female presents to urgent care with swelling of a mass in her neck for the past 4 weeks.*

INTRODUCTION TO COMPLAINT

There are numerous lymph nodes throughout the body. A few areas are palpable, namely, the submandibular, axillary, and inguinal regions. Most enlarged nodes are benign. If a node is larger than 1 cm, it should be considered potentially abnormal and if it is 3 cm or greater, suspect neoplastic (cancer) disease.

Common causes of enlarged lymph nodes are infections and malignancies. When a node is enlarged due to an infection it is called a "reactive node."

Bacterial Infections

- AIDS or HIV infection
- Mononucleosis
- Toxoplasmosis
- Secondary syphilis
- AIDS-related complex

Malignancy

- Non-Hodgkin's lymphoma
- Hodgkin's disease in advanced stages
- Leukemia

HISTORY OF COMPLAINT

Symptomatology

Ask about the following characteristics of each symptom using open-ended questions:

- Chronology
- Current situation (improving or deteriorating)
- Location
- Radiation
- Quality
- Timing (frequency, duration)
- Severity
- Precipitating and aggravating factors
- Relieving factors
- Associated symptoms
- Effects on daily activities

- Previous diagnosis of similar episodes
- Previous treatments
- Efficacy of previous treatments

Directed Questions to Ask

- Can you remember how long this swelling of the node has been present?
- Can you describe the way it feels? Is it hard, rubbery, or soft?
- Has it changed in size, shape, or consistency over time?
- Has it been tender?
- Have you had any fever, chills, sweats, or weight loss?
- Have you felt more fatigued than usual?
- Have you had any bruising or abnormal bleeding?
- Have you had more than the usual number of illnesses lately?
- Have you had a sore throat, nasal congestion, or eye infection?
- Have you had any problems with your teeth or dental infections?
- Have you had sex with men, women, or both? Do you practice safe sex?
- Have had any sexually transmitted infections such as herpes?
  Do you have any open sores?
- Do you have a cat or any other animals? Have they bitten or scratched you?

Assessment: Cardinal Signs and Symptoms

Location of the node	Questions
Submandibular	Is there a sore throat or infection in the mouth?
Cervical anterior aspect	Head, neck, or throat infection? Do you have fever, chills, sweats, or weight loss?
Cervical posterior	Have you had any localized infections of the skin in the area of the enlarged node? Infection of the scalp, mononucleosis, toxoplasmosis? Any recent contact with others who are ill? Do you have a cat?
Right supraclavicular	Do you have difficulty swallowing? Have you been a smoker? Do you have a cough?
Left supraclavicular	Do you have heartburn, lack of appetite, change in bowel habits? Have you been screened for colon cancer? When was your last Pap smear?
Epitrochlear	Do you have sores anywhere? Have you injured your hand? Do you have a cat or has any animal scratched or bitten you?
Inguinal	Do you have any open sores on the genital area? Do you have any recent injury or infection to the leg or feet?
Preauricular	Do you have pain in the eyes, discharge? Do you have pain in the ears? Do you have nasal discharge or pain?

Medical History: General

- Medical history: Acute and chronic illness
- Family history: Any history of cancer, sarcoidosis, TB, or autoimmune disease
- Social history, including exposures to carcinogens, tobacco, and alcohol; any pets
- Medications especially Dilantin, which may cause a reactive node

Medical History: Specific to Complaint

- Previous history of enlarged lymph nodes
- Autoimmune disorders

PHYSICAL EXAMINATION

Vital Signs

- Temperature
- Pulse
- Respirations
- Blood pressure

General Appearance

- Overall appearance
- Any signs of obvious distress
- Color of skin
- Skin tugor
- Hygiene

Head, Eyes, Ears, Nose, Throat (HEENT)
- Examine HEENT to determine presence of infectious process especially noting dental, ears, and throat infection or abnormality

Neck
- Palpate all lymph nodes and describe size, shape, mobility, and texture

Cardiac
- Listen to heart for rate, rhythm, the presence of murmurs

Lungs
- Listen to all lobes
- Note any abnormality or diminished breath sounds that may indicate a pleural effusion

Abdomen
- Observe for enlarged abdominal girth indicating the presence of fluid
- Palpate for tenderness
- Evaluate the liver and spleen for any increase in size
- Palpate for abnormal masses

Genitourinary
- Perform a pelvic or genital examination if lesions are in the inguinal area

Rectal
- Perform a rectal examination if lesions are in the left supraclavicular or inguinal area

Skin
- Observe for jaundice, purpura, and petechial or abnormal rashes; observe for redness, scratches, or open wounds

Extremities
- Observe for edema of lower extremities, clubbing of nails, or deformity

CASE STUDY
History

Question	Response
How long has swelling of the node been present?	*At least 4 weeks, maybe more*
Did it occur all of the sudden?	*Yes, just woke up with it*
Can you describe the way it feels?	*It is just hard, no pain, just hard*
Has it changed at all?	*Yes, it is twice the size it was last month*
Have you had any fevers or chills?	*No, never*
Have you had any sweats?	*On occasion I do sweat at night*
Have you lost any weight?	*I wish, no, I eat well and my weight is good*
Have you been more fatigued?	*A little bit, but I watch the grandbaby now*
Have you had any abnormal bruising?	*No, have not noticed that*
Have you been sick a lot this year?	*Yes, I watch the baby, so I am always sick*
Have you had a recent dental problem	*No, I have dentures now*
Have you had a sore throat?	*Yes, about 2 months ago, another cold*
Is it sore now?	*No, it is fine*
Have you had any sinus pain?	*No, nothing hurts*
Have you had nasal discharge?	*Not now, that cleared up months ago*
Do you have problems swallowing?	*No, I eat everything*
Do you have any cats or animals?	*No, not now, our tabby died 6 months ago*
Have you had any scalp infections?	*I do get dandruff now and then*
Is there anything else you would like to add?	*No, you have been quite thorough*

Physical Examination Findings
- VITAL SIGNS: 98.8°F, respiratory rate (RR) 20, heart rate (HR) 72, BP 124/72
- GENERAL APPEARANCE: well-developed, petite female in no distress
- EYES: no injection, anicteric, pupils equal, round, and reactive to light and accommodation (PERRLA), extraocular movements intact

- NOSE: nares are patent; no edema or exudate of turbinates
- MOUTH: teeth and gums are in good repair (gums are pink; teeth are without decay); no oral lesions
- PHARYNX: tonsils not enlarged; no redness, exudate
- NECK: right tonsillar node is 3 × 3 cm, hard, and fixed; no other anterior or posterior nodes are enlarged; neck is supple; thyroid is not enlarged
- LYMPH: axillary, epitrochlear, and inguinal nodes are not palpable
- CHEST: lungs are clear in all fields; heart S1 S2 no murmur, gallop, or rub
- ABDOMEN: soft, obese, nontender without mass or organomegaly
- SKIN: no rashes

DIFFERENTIAL DIAGNOSIS

Differential Diagnosis	Oral or Pharyngeal Infection	Non-Hodgkin's Lymphoma	Mononucleosis
Onset	Gradual or sudden	Sudden	Gradual or sudden
Dental pain or sore throat	Yes	No	+ or −
Fever	Yes	No	Yes
Weight loss	No	Later stages	No
Night sweats	If fever	Yes	If fever
Fatigue	+ or −	Later stages	Yes
Exposed to cat	No	No	No
Node	Tender, rubbery mobile	Hard, tender, nonmobile	Tender, firm posterior and anterior

DIAGNOSTIC EXAMINATION

Examination	Procedure Code	Cost	Results
Complete blood count (CBC)	85025	$75	CBC The CBC typically has several parameters that are created from an automated cell counter. The most relevant are: • White blood count (WBC): White blood cells protect the body against infection. When there is an infection present, the WBC rises very quickly. WBC includes a differential white count.

(continued)

Examination	Procedure Code	Cost	Results

Complete blood count (CBC) (*continued*)			• WBC differential:
			  ▪ Neurtophils: The most abundant of the white blood cells increase rapidly to areas of injury and infection.
			  ▪ Eosinophils: Are active during allergic or parasitic illnesses.
			  ▪ Basophils: Will increase during the healing process.
			  ▪ Monocytes: Are the second defense mechanism against bacterial and inflammatory illnesses. Slower to respond than neutrophils but are bigger and can ingest larger organisms or foreign bodies.
			  ▪ Lymphocytes: Increase after chronic bacterial and viral infections.
			• Red blood cells (RBCs): Carry O_2 from the lungs to the body.
			• Hematocrit: A measure of the number of RBCs in a space.
			• Hemoglobin: Protein substance that carries oxygen and gives RBCs their color. It is a good measure to determine the ability of the blood to carry oxygen throughout the body.
			• Mean corpuscular volume (MCV): Determines the volume of the RBCs.
			• Mean corpuscular hemoglobin (MCH): Shows the amount of hemoglobin contained in the average RBC
			• Mean corpuscular hemoglobin concentration (MCHC): Measures the concentration of the hemoglobin in an average RBC.
			• Platelets: The platelets play an important role in blood clotting. If there are too few platelets, uncontrolled bleeding can occur. If there are too many, a blood clot can form in the artery.

Complete metabolic panel (CMP)	80053	$49	• Glucose level: Elevated levels are seen in patients with diabetes, adrenal gland dysfunction, stress, burns, and most important, infection. • Creatinine clearance: Decreased levels could be an indicator of renal impairment. • Alkaline phosphatase, alanine aminotransferase, aspartate aminotransferase: These are all diagnostic tests that indicate how the liver is functioning.

CLINICAL DECISION MAKING

Case Study Analysis

Sudden onset of a large 3 × 3 cm nontender, hard, nonmobile lymph node localized to the anterior cervical chain. Patient complains of occasional night sweats but denies fever or chills. Rule out pharyngitis, dental caries and abscess, and lesions.

Diagnosis: *Lymphadenopathy*

FURTHER READING

Goroll, A. H., May, L., & Mulley, A. G., Jr. (1998). *Primary care medicine* (2nd ed.). Philadelphia, PA: Lippincott Williams & Wilkins.

EYE DISCHARGE

Case Presentation: *A 6-year-old female presents with left eye redness and crusting for 2 days. She arrives in the company of her mother.*

INTRODUCTION TO COMPLAINT

- Multiple conditions can lead to eye discharge
- Viral or bacterial conjunctivitis, also known as "pinkeye"; this is the most common type
- In newborns, ophthalmia neonatorum can, if not treated, lead to permanent scarring and blindness
- Viral conjunctivitis is often accompanied by an upper respiratory infection (URI)
- Viral herpes zoster, which, if not closely monitored and treated, can lead to blindness
- Allergic conjunctivitis: generally affects both eyes and is accompanied by other allergic symptoms, such as rhinitis
- Dacryostenosis is an obstruction of the nasolacrimal duct due to incomplete formation or cyst formation within; it can lead to tearing and matting in newborns
- Eyelid condition, such as blepharitis, ingrown lashes, hordoleum, or chalazion
- Injury: corneal abrasion or ulcer can lead to excessive tearing and mucoid discharge, with the possibility of superinfection

HISTORY OF COMPLAINT

Symptomatology

Ask about the following characteristics of each symptom using open-ended questions:

- Onset
- Location
- Duration, timing, frequency
- Character of the discharge or presence of pain
- Associated symptoms
- Aggravating factors
- Alleviating factors
- Effect on daily activities

Directed Questions to Ask

- One eye or both?
- Describe the discharge. Is it mucoid, pus-like, tearing, crusting? Is there any matting of the eyelashes?
- Is it worsening, improving, or remaining stable?
- Any recent illness or associated symptoms?
- Rate your discomfort on a pain scale. Is it persistent or intermittent?
- Does anything make it better (keeping eyes closed, darkening the room) or worse (light exposure, etc.)?
- Do you wear contacts?

Assessment: Cardinal Signs and Symptoms

General
- Fever, chills, malaise, pain

Eyes
- Visual disturbance, pain/itching/foreign body sensation, eyelid involvement

Head, Ears, Nose, Throat (HENT)
- Headache, photophobia, visual disturbance, runny nose, congestion, sneezing, facial swelling

Respiratory
- Cough, wheezing, dypnea

Skin
- Rashes, local swelling

Lymph
- Swollen nodes

Medical History: General

- MEDICAL HISTORY: medical conditions (treated and untreated), surgeries, allergies, current medications, and over-the-counter therapies
- FAMILY MEDICAL HISTORY: medical conditions in close, blood-related relatives
- SOCIAL HISTORY: substance use (drugs/alcohol), leisure activities, recent travel/exposures

Medical History: Specific to Complaint

- Matted lashes
- Decreased visual acuity
- Tearing of the eyes
- Stringy discharge

PHYSICAL EXAMINATION
Vital Signs

- Heart rate (HR)
- Respiratory rate (RR)

- Blood pressure (BP)
- Oxygen saturation (SpO$_2$)
- Temperature
- Pain scale

General Appearance

- Calm or distressed

Visual Acuity
- Corrected with glasses if patient has baseline diminished acuity
- Measure each eye in isolation as well as both together

HENT
- Lesions (especially surrounding eyes, ear canals, tip of nose)
- Rhinorrhea
- Boggy turbinates or hyperemia
- Allergic shiners
- Local swelling or swelling over nasolacrimal duct

Eyes
- Unilateral or bilateral
- Pupils equal, round, and reactive to light and accommodation (PERRLA)
- Extraocular movements
- Eyelid involvement
- Evert eyelids for examination
- Matting of lashes
- Conjunctival injection
- Ciliary flush
- Fluorescein uptake (extent, location, pattern)
- Peripheral vision
- Corneal opacity/cloudiness

Neck
- Lymphadenopathy

CASE STUDY
History

Question	Response
Which eye is bothering her? Or is it both?	*Left eye*
Can you describe the drainage for me?	*There is a stringy discharge during the day. It's crusty, and gets on her eyelashes at night.*
When did it begin?	*She woke up with it yesterday morning*

Question	Response
Has she had any injuries or exposures?	*No*
Is it worsening, improving, or remaining stable?	*It's worst in the mornings, and it seems to be worse today than yesterday*
Has she had any recent illness?	*Upper respiratory infection (URI). She's had a runny nose for a week. No fever.*
Are there any associated symptoms?	*Just the runny nose; itchy throat*
Has she complained of eye pain?	*No, she hasn't complained at all, she just keeps rubbing and wiping it*
Does she have any medical problems that you are aware of?	*She was premature (2 weeks) and she had a hernia repair. Nothing else significant.*
Do you have any concerns for her vision?	*I don't think so*
How does it feel? Does it hurt? Is it itchy?	*Patient: It scratches me! (rubbing eyes)*

Physical Examination Findings

- VITAL SIGNS: temperature 98.6°F (oral), HR 90, RR 20
- GENERAL APPEARANCE: alert, very active, and friendly
- VISUAL ACUITY: oculus dexter (OD) 20/40; oculus sinister (OS) 20/40-1; oculus uterque (OU) 20/40
- HENT: no rashes or lesions; moderate mucoid rhinitis; tympanic membrane dullness bilaterally
- EYES: PERRLA 3+, extraocular movement intact (EOMI); fluorescein examination—no uptake, except for slight mucoid drainage to inner canthus; left eye—both eyelids everted for examination; mild injection in left eye, no ciliary flush; minimal crusting noted to lower lateral lashes; no lid lesions or swelling; rubbing eyes frequently throughout examination
- NECK/LYMPH: supple, no lymphadenopathy
- CARDIOVASCULAR: regular rate and rhythm (RRR), no murmurs
- LUNGS: clear to auscultation (CTA), good air entry bilaterally, no respiratory distress
- SKIN: warm and dry with good color; no rashes noted

DIFFERENTIAL DIAGNOSIS

Differential Diagnosis	Bacterial Conjunctivitis	Viral Conjunctivitis	Allergic Conjunctivitis	Dacryostenosis	Injury	Gonorrhea/ Chlamydia	Blepharitis
History	Possible known history of exposure, especially among children	Often associated with URI symptoms but may occur in isolation	Possible known or suspected exposure; consider environmental as well as topical (makeup, etc.) or aerosolized agents	Noted at or shortly after birth	Often recalls specific incident of foreign body to the eye or irritant exposure	Born vaginally to mother with active chlamydia/ gonorrhea infection or no prenatal care; can also be self-inoculated by touching infected genitals and then eyes	May have concurrent history of seborrheic dermatitis
Age	Most common in children, can occur at any age	Most common in children, can occur at any age	Usually adult onset	Most common in newborns, usually resolves within first year of life	Any	Neonate (generally 5–14 days after delivery), or concurrent genital infection	Any
Discomfort	Irritation	Itching, gritty sensation, or burning	Itching, gritty sensation, or burning		Pain or foreign body sensation	Irritation	Irritation
Discharge	Copious purulent; may be white, yellow, or green with morning matting; accumulates in corners of the eye and on lid margins	Mucoid and crusting	Tearing and mucoid (stringy)	Chronic or intermittent tearing, often eyelash matting; tears/mucoid discharge with palpation of lacrimal duct	Tearing	Can begin as watery discharge, progresses to mucopurulent	Crusting at lid margins, or greasy flakes

(continued)

Differential Diagnosis	Bacterial Conjunctivitis	Viral Conjunctivitis	Allergic Conjunctivitis	Dacryostenosis	Injury	Gonorrhea/ Chlamydia	Blepharitis
Rhinitis	No	Common	Common		No	No	No
Unilateral or bilateral	Unilateral or bilateral	Often unilateral at first and proceeds to bilateral in 1 to 2 days	Bilateral (unless unilateral direct contact with irritant)	Usually unilateral	Usually unilateral	Bilateral in ophthalmia neonatorum; unilateral or bilateral in the adult	Bilateral
Eyelid involvement	No	No	Sometimes			Yes	Yes, reddened, often with dry flaking skin; waxy secretions may occur at meibomian gland openings
Other	Tarsal conjunctivae injected	Tarsal conjunctivae injected	Tarsal conjunctivae injected	May find swelling of skin overlying nasolacrimal duct	Special attention in patients wearing contact lenses	Eye discharge may become blood stained and pseudo-membrane may form; referral is indicated	Inflamma-tion at lid margins; tear film irregularity

DIAGNOSTIC EXAMINATION

Examination	Procedure Code	Cost	Results	Notes
Rapid adenovirus test	87809QW	$15	Positive = viral conjunctivitis	An inconclusive test that does not help with diagnosis; acceptable sensitivity and specificity (Sambursky et al., 2013); can help prevent antibiotic misuse
Fluorescein examination	92225–92260	NA	Uptake indicates disruption in corneal surface	
Visual acuity	99172	NA	Red flag: gross loss of vision	Test corrected vision if possible
Culture	87040–87255	$35	Positive = bacterial conjunctivitis Rapid onset	Must be collected from everted eyelid, simple exudate collection insufficient because sample must include conjunctival epithelial cells

CLINICAL DECISION MAKING

Case Study Analysis

The advanced practice nurse (APN) performs the assessment and physical examination on the patient and describes 36 hours' duration of unilateral pink eye with crusting. Left eye exhibits mild but diffuse injection, including injection of the tarsal conjunctiva. The child also exhibits a copiously runny nose. Her history and examination are notable for the absence of periorbital edema or eye pain. On fluorescein examination there is no uptake of dye to suggest a corneal abrasion. Visual acuity 20/20.

> **Diagnosis:** *Viral conjunctivitis*

- At times, a patient will present with a confusing history regarding the nature of the discharge that does not effectively point toward a viral or bacterial cause
- Swab for adenovirus can be helpful
- Those who present with classic viral conjunctivitis require good hand washing, gentle and frequent cleansing of crusting, and the passage of time
- Excessive itching can often be improved with the use of artificial tears (or eye lubricant ointment) for comfort or, if needed, topical ophthalmic antihistamine/decongestant drops
- Antibiotics are not indicated

- Anticipatory guidance should include that it may worsen over the next few days and/or spread to the other eye, and recovery may take 2 weeks or more a cool compress may provide comfort in the interim, along with gentle eyelid cleansing from the inner canthus outward along closed eyelids

FURTHER READING

Sambursky, R., Trattler, W., Tauber, S., Starr, C., Friedberg, M., Boland, T., . . . Luchs, J. (2013). Sensitivity and specificity of the AdenoPlus test for diagnosing adenoviral conjunctivitis. *JAMA Ophthalmology, 131*(1), 17–21.

EYE PAIN

Case Presentation: *A 74-year-old man is complaining of left eye pain that began when he woke up from a nap. The pain worsened rapidly and he has a headache, nausea, and blurred vision in the affected eye.*

INTRODUCTION TO COMPLAINT

Primary causes of eye pain are:

- Ocular trauma
  - Corneal abrasion
- Infection
  - Bacterial conjunctivitis
- Inflammation
  - Iritis/uveitis
  - Scleritis
- Increased intraocular pressure (IOP)
  - Acute angle glaucoma

HISTORY OF COMPLAINT

Symptomatology

Ask about the following characteristics of each symptom using open-ended questions:

- Onset
- Duration, timing, frequency of pain
- Location
- Character of pain
- Associated symptoms
- Aggravating factors
- Alleviating factors
- Effect on daily activities

Directed Questions to Ask

- Can you tell me about your eye pain?
- Was the onset sudden or gradual?
- Where exactly in the eye is your pain?
- Are both eyes involved or is the pain only in your left eye?
- How would you describe your pain: is it like stabbing, throbbing, burning, sharp, aching pain or a "something in my eye" feeling?

- Is your pain continuous or intermittent and, if it is intermittent, how long does it last?
- If 0 is no pain and 10 is the worst pain you have ever had, what number is this pain?
- Is the pain worse when you move your eyes?
- Is there anything that precipitates or aggravates your symptoms?
- Is there anything that alleviates your pain?
- Did something get into your eye?
- How is your vision? Is it blurred or do you feel blind spots that suddenly appear?
- Do you have photophobia or double vision?
- Is the eye dry or watering?
- Do you have eye itching?
- What other symptoms do you have?
- What concerns you most about the pain?
- Did you ever have this type of eye pain before? If yes, what was the treatment you received?

Assessment: Cardinal Signs and Symptoms

Head
- Headache? Unilateral or bilateral? Throbbing or aching
- On a scale of 0 to 10, if 0 is no pain and 10 is the worst pain you ever had, how bad is the pain?
- Is pain continuous or intermittent?

Nose and Sinuses
- Facial tenderness, pain, or pressure
- Nasal/sinus congestion or stuffiness
- Nasal congestion on one or both sides
- Loss of smell

Ears
- How is your hearing
- Any history of hearing loss
- Ear ache or pain in the ear

Other Associated Symptoms
- Fever
- Cough
- Nausea or vomiting
- Anxious or stressed

Medical History: General

- Medical conditions like diabetes, high blood pressure, high cholesterol, tuberculosis (TB), or any previous herpes infections like cytomegalovirus (CMV)
- Stroke or family history of stroke or other neurological problems
- Chronic headache or migraine
- Heart problems or history of cardiovascular disease like heart failure, heart attack, or cardiovascular occlusion
- Breathing or respiratory problems in the past
- Surgeries in the past
- Allergies to foods, medications, or plants
- Seasonal allergy
- Sinusitis
- Current use of medications, including prescription medications
- Use of over-the-counter medications
- Use of any herbal preparations or traditional therapies

Medical History: Specific to Complaint

- Frequent eye pain or infections
- Diagnosis of glaucoma, retinopathy, or retinal hemorrhage
- Trauma to eyes
- Past eye surgery
- Exposure to chemicals

PHYSICAL EXAMINATION

Vital Signs

- Temperature
- Respiratory rate
- Heart rate
- Blood pressure (BP)

General Appearance

- Overall appearance
- Any signs of obvious distress
- Skin color, turgor, capillary refill response
- Difficulty with gait or balance

Head
- Inspect for lesions or trauma
- Inspect for involuntary movement

Eyes
- Inspect for any redness in eyes
- Any change in vision
- Photophobia

Ear
- Hearing

Nose and Sinus
- Drainage and edema
- Inspect for tenderness

Neurologic
- Mental status
- Cranial nerves
- Motor system
- Reflexes

CASE STUDY

History

Question	Response
Can you tell me about your eye pain?	*I can't open my eyes, it hurts so bad*
Was the onset sudden or gradual?	*It was sudden and I'm scared*
Where exactly in the eye is your pain?	*It seems to come from inside my eye*

Question	*Response*
Are both eyes involved or is it only in your left eye?	*Only my left eye hurts*
Is your pain radiating to anywhere else?	*Yes, to the back of my eye*
How would you describe your pain?	*It's like a hot poker in the center of my eye*
Is your pain continuous or intermittent?	*It is continuous*
On a scale of 0 to 10, with 10 being the worst pain you have ever had, what number is this pain?	*13, the pain is so bad that I don't think I can take it anymore*
Is the pain worse when you move your eyes?	*No*
Is there anything that precipitates or aggravates your symptoms?	*Light increases the pain*
Is there anything that alleviates your pain?	*Nothing seems to help*
Did something get into your eye?	*No*
How is your vision: Is it blurred or do you see blind spots?	*I think I can see well*
Do you have double vision?	*No*
Is the eye dry or watering?	*No*
Does your eye itch?	*No*
What other symptoms do you have?	*I have a constant headache. This pain affects my thinking.*
What concerns you most about the pain?	*The pain is so bad I'm afraid*
Did you ever have this type of eye pain before?	*No*

Physical Examination Findings

- VITAL SIGNS: BP 135/82, pulse 92 regular, respiratory rate 22 regular
- GENERAL APPEARANCE: appears distressed and in pain; difficulty answering questions and keeping his eyes open; skin pale and sweaty
- HEAD: free of lesions or evidence of trauma; normocephalic, normal hair distribution; brows symetrical
- EYES: clear; patient complains of blurred vision and visual acuity test reveals the ability to detect only hand movements; patient unable to identify numbers and letters on distance charts or near cards; cornea and scleral injection and ciliary flush are present; the obviously edematous and cloudy cornea obscures funduscopic examination; extremely hard to examine left eye due to patient's complaint of pain; increased IOP (normal limit, 10–20 mmHg) and ischemia result in pain on eye movement, a mid-dilated nonreactive pupil, and a firm globe

DIFFERENTIAL DIAGNOSIS

Differential Diagnosis	Cerebrovascular Accident	Uveitis	Traumatic Hyphema	Acute Angle Closure Glaucoma	Migraine
Onset	Sudden	Gradual/abrupt	Abrupt	Sudden	Sudden
Pain	Pain	Aching	+	Severe	Severe
Vision loss	Blurred/loss	Blurred	+	Blurred	Blurred
Bleeding eye	–	+	+	–	–
Light sensitivity	Photophobia	Photophobia	–	–	Photophobia
Numbness/ weakness/paralysis	Yes	–	–	–	–
Pupil	–	–	–	Nonreactive	–
Headache	Severe	Rare	–	Severe	Severe
Nausea/vomiting	Common	Rare	Common	Yes	Yes
Intraocular pressure	–	Rare	Common	High > 21	–
Red eye	–	Common	–	Yes	–
Floaters	–	Common	Rare	Rare	–
Photophobia	–	–	–	–	Common

DIAGNOSTIC EXAMINATION

Eye Examination	Procedure Code	Cost	Results
Physical examination	99397	$250	• Right eye examination: fixed mid-dilated nonreactive pupil • Nonreactive pupils also can be a sign of intracranial injury • Unable to examine left eye
Tonometry	89.11	Cost varies depending on age and comorbid factors	• Tonometry measures the pressure within the eyes. Most glaucoma cases are diagnosed with pressure exceeding 20 mmHg. In IOP, it will be more than 21 mmHg in most of the cases. • This examination helps to determine the angle where the iris meets the cornea • If the angle is narrow and closed, then it is closed-angle glaucoma

(continued)

Eye Examination	Procedure Code	Cost	Results
Perimetry	92083	Cost varies depending on age and comorbid factors	• Perimetry is a visual field test that determines how much of the vision is affected • Checks peripheral vision
CT scan of the brain	70450	$1250	• Visualizes components of the brain, size, location, and integrity

CLINICAL DECISION MAKING

Case Study Analysis

The provider performs the physical examination on the patient and finds the following data: sudden onset of left eye pain, worsening eye pain 30 minutes after the complaint, with headache, nausea, and blurred vision. The reaction to light of the left pupil is sluggish compared to the right eye. Unable to examine left eye.

> **Diagnosis:** *Acute angle closure glaucoma*

Pressure inside the eye rises suddenly. Symptoms include severe eye pain, nausea and vomiting, headache, and decreased vision. These symptoms are an emergency and need immediate treatment to prevent blindness.

FURTHER READING

Haini, M. H. H. (n.d.). *Ocular history taking.* Retrieved from http://www.fastbleep.com/medical-notes/surgery/20/46/706

Rhoads, J., & Petersen, S. (2013). *Advanced health assessment and diagnostic reasoning* (2nd ed.). Sudbury, MA: Jones & Bartlett.

Thomas, R., Loibl, K., & Parikh, R. (2011). How to assess a patient with glaucoma. *Indian Journal of Ophthalmology, 59*(Suppl. 1), S43–S52. doi:10.4103/0301-4738.73688

Thomas, R., & Parikh, R. S. (2006). Evaluation of a glaucoma patient. *Community Eye Health, 19*(59), 36–37.

EYE REDNESS

Case Presentation: *A 12-year-old female patient complains of red left eye and edematous eyelids. Her mother states the child complains of "sand in my left eye."*

INTRODUCTION TO COMPLAINT

Red eyes are caused by swollen or dilated blood vessels on the sclera. Red eyes can be accompanied by itching, pain, discharge, swelling, and visual acuity changes.

Viral Infections

- Red eyes can be caused by viral illness, such as adenovirus, piconavirus, rhinovirus, and herpes simplex virus.
- Viral conjunctivitis has a gradual onset with unilateral symptoms and no pain.
- Visual acuity is intact.
- Watery discharge is apparent.
- Blepharitis is the most common cause of inflammation of the eyelid. It is bilateral and associated with conjunctivitis.

Bacterial Infections

- A bacterial infection can also cause red eyes.
- *Staphylococcus aureus, Streptococcus pneumonia*, group A *Streptococcus, Haemophilus influenza*, and *Neisseria gonorrhoeae* are the most common causes of bacterial conjunctivitis (Dains, Baumann, & Scheibel, 2012).
- Bacterial conjunctivitis has a gradual onset, unilateral early, bilateral late; scratchy (no pain); photophobia (not generally present).
- The thick crusty discharge that is present in bacterial infections may cause "blurry" vision.
- Blepharitis can also be caused by bacterial infections.

Irritants and Injuries

- Trauma to the eye can also cause red eyes.
- Improper contact lens care can cause red eyes, which can be symptoms of keratitis or fungal eye infections.
- Subconjuctival hemorrhage can cause the eye to appear red because of the broken blood vessels present in the conjunctival tissues.

Allergic Conjunctivitis

- Allergic conjunctivitis is a chronic and seasonal condition that can cause the eyes to be bilaterally red and itchy. It is painless and causes a mucoid discharge (Dains, Baumann, & Scheibel, 2012).

HISTORY OF COMPLAINT
Symptomatology

Ask about the following characteristics of each symptom using open-ended questions:

- Chronology
- Current situation (improving or deteriorating)
- Location
- Radiation
- Quality
- Timing (frequency, duration)
- Severity
- Precipitating and aggravating factors
- Relieving factors
- Associated symptoms
- Effects on daily activities
- Previous diagnosis of similar episodes
- Previous treatments
- Efficacy of previous treatments

Directed Questions to Ask

- When did you first notice the redness and tearing?
- Was the onset gradual or sudden?
- Do you have any known allergies?
- Have your symptoms gotten worse since you first noticed them?
- What symptom did you notice first and how did your symptoms progress?
- Have you been around anyone who has had an eye infection that you were aware of?
- Do you have any pain in either eye?
- Have you had any other symptoms other than the redness, tearing, swelling, and "sand in eye feeling"? Such as nausea, vomiting, sore throat, fever, coughs, and so on.
- Do you have any thick discharge or crusting of either eye?
- Have your symptoms affected your ability to see well?
- Have you injured your eye?
- Do you wear contacts?

Assessment: Cardinal Signs and Symptoms
Head, Ears, Nose, Throat
- Sore throat recently
- Runny nose
- Sneezing
- Enlarged lymph nodes
- Itchy eyes
- Crust in eyes

Medical History: General

- Medical conditions and surgeries
- Allergies
- Medication currently used and over the counter meds currently used
- Herbal or traditional therapies

Medical History: Specific to Complaint

- Frequent eye infections
- Glasses or contacts
- Last eye examination
- Double vision, blurred vision, spots, specks, flashing lights

PHYSICAL EXAMINATION

Vital Signs

- Temperature
- Pulse
- Respiration
- SpO_2 (oxygen saturation)
- Blood pressure

General Appearance

- Apparent state of health
- Appearance of comfort or distress
- Color
- Nutritional status
- State of hydration
- Hygiene

Eye Inspection

- Position and alignment of eyes
- Eyebrows: noticing their quantity and distribution, scaliness of underlying skin
- Eyelids: width, edema, color, lesions, condition, and direction of eyelashes, adequacy with which the eyelids close
- Lacrimal apparatus: inspect lacrimal gland and sac for swelling, excessive tearing, or dryness
- Conjunctiva and sclera
- Cornea and lens
- Iris
- Pupils

Palpation

- Tenderness, enlargement, mobility, contour, and consistency of nodes and masses
- Nodes: pre- and postauricle, occipital, tonsillar, submandibular, submental

CASE STUDY

History

Question	Response
When did you first notice the redness and tearing?	*Three days ago*
Was the onset gradual or sudden?	*Gradual*
Do you have any known allergies?	*None known*
Have your symptoms gotten worse since you first noticed them?	*Yes*

Question	*Response*
What symptoms did you notice first and how did your symptoms progress?	*Redness when I first woke up this morning then pain due to gritty feeling*
Have you been around anyone who has had an eye infection that you were aware of?	*Yes, my little girl*
Do you have any pain in either eye?	*No, just feels like I have something in my eye*
Have you had any other symptoms other than the redness, tearing, swelling, and "sand in eye feeling"? Such as nausea, vomiting, sore throat, fever, coughs…	*No*
Do you have any thick discharge or crusting of either eye?	*Yes, crust around my left eye, difficult to open it up this morning*
Have your symptoms affected your ability to see well?	*Yes. With difficulty opening up my eye when the crust builds up*
Have you injured your eye?	*No*
Do you wear contacts?	*No*

Physical Examination Findings

- VITAL SIGNS: 98.2°F, respiratory rate (RR) 18, heart rate (HR) 78, weight 110 lbs
- GENERAL APPEARANCE: well-developed, healthy, 12 years old
- EYES: very red sclera with dried, crusty exudates; unable to open eyes in the morning—with the left being worse than the right
- EARS: no edema, no exudates
- NOSE: no edema, no exudates, no boggy turbinates
- MOUTH: no edema, no exudates
- PHARYNX: moderately large, no exudates
- NECK: no edema, no palpable nodes; neck is supple; thyroid not enlarged

DIFFERENTIAL DIAGNOSIS

Differential Diagnosis	Bacterial Conjunctivitis	Blepharitis	Viral Conjunctivitis	Allergic Conjunctivitis
Both eyes	Yes	Yes	No	Yes
Sclera	Red	Red	Red	Red
Itchiness	Yes	Yes	Yes	Yes
Exudate	Yes	Yes	Yes	Yes
Epiphora	Yes	Yes	Yes	Yes
Boggy turbinates	No	No	No	Yes

DIAGNOSTIC EXAMINATIONS

Examinations	Procedure Code	Cost	Results
Vision screening	V72.0	$50 to $100	Determine visual acuity
Eye examination	V72.0	$50 to $100	Examine corneal light reflex, accommodation, stabismus, and extraocular movements
Eye culture and sensitivity	372.3	$35 to $55	Identify whether bacteria is present
Wood's lamp test	V72.0	Part of the eye examination	Assess for corneal abrasion
Transillumination of the sinus cavity	V72.0	Part of the physical examination fee, which varies between providers	Assess for consolidation of the sinuses

CLINICAL DECISION MAKING

Case Study Analysis

The advanced practice nurse performs the assessment and physical examination on the patients and finds the following pertinent positives: bilateral redness of sclera, exudates, profuse tearing, and edematous eyelids. Patient complains of "sand" in left eye. The pertinent negatives are no loss of vision, history of trauma, or severe eye pain.

> ***Diagnosis:*** *Bacterial conjunctivitis*

It is important to remember that eye infections are treated empirically with antibiotic eye drops. It is not necessary to culture the eye discharge. The symptoms usually resolve in 2 to 3 days. Persistent redness, vision change, or pain warrants immediate referral.

FURTHER READING

Chou, B. (2013). *Eye infections, including bacterial, fungal, and viral.* Retrieved from http://www
.allaboutvision.com/conditions/eye-infections.htm#type

Dains, J., Baumann, L., & Scheibel, P. (2012). *Advanced health assessment and clinical diagnosis in primary care* (5th ed.). St. Louis, MO: Mosby.

Heiting, G., & Palombi, J. (2013). *Eye exam costs and when to have an eye exam.* Retrieved from http://
www.allaboutvision.com/eye-exam/preparing.htm

Rhoads, J., & Petersen, S. (2013). *Advanced health assessment and diagnostic reasoning* (2nd ed.). Sudbury, MA: Jones & Bartlett.

FATIGUE

Case Presentation: *A 23-year-old Caucasian single mother of two (ages 4 and 2) presents to the clinic complaining of persistent fatigue. She is in a stable dating relationship with a childhood schoolmate, works 3 days a week as a medical assistant, and has been taking night classes toward getting into nursing school.*

INTRODUCTION TO COMPLAINT

Fatigue as a lone presenting problem is vague and can be a frustrating problem to assess. It is important to note the duration of the fatigue, as the longer it is present without any other associated symptom, the more likely it is to be psychogenic. Almost all illnesses are capable of causing fatigue. The differential diagnosis is broad and falls into the following general categories:

- Psychologic
- Endocrine
- Pharmacologic
- Cardiopulmonary
- Hematologic
- Oncologic
- Infectious

HISTORY OF COMPLAINT

Symptomatology

Ask about the following characteristics of each symptom using open-ended questions:

- Onset
- Course
- Preceding symptoms
- Sleep habits

Directed Questions to Ask

- When did it begin? (less than 1 month ago, more than 1 month ago, 6 months ago or longer) Was the onset sudden or gradual?
- How often does it occur? How long does it last? Is it improving, worsening, stable, or intermittent?
- Were there any suspected precipitating events? (trauma, exposure, life change, etc.)
- Have you had any recent or frequent illnesses? Any recent sore throat?

- What makes it better or worse? What have you tried so far to improve your fatigue?
- Are there any associated symptoms? (insomnia, fever, vomiting/diarrhea, persistent sadness, sleep deprivation, appetite change, suicidal ideation, weight loss/gain, night sweats, skin/hair changes, exercise intolerance, dyspnea, swollen glands, memory loss, muscle weakness, palpitations, etc.)
- How has it affected your activities of daily living? (missed work days, relational changes, grooming, family adjustments made, etc.)
- Can you describe the quality of your sleep? (restful, fractured) How many hours do you sleep at one time? Any night shifts? Naps? How long does it take to get to sleep? What is your nighttime routine?
- What medications are you taking? Have there been any recent changes? (obtain information on all regular and medications taken as needed, including over-the-counter medications and especially any changes around time of onset of fatigue)

Assessment: Cardinal Signs and Symptoms

Address the following specifics in addition to the above questions:

- MEDICAL HISTORY: medical conditions (treated and untreated), surgeries, allergies, current medications, and over-the-counter therapies
- FAMILY MEDICAL HISTORY: medical conditions in close, blood-related relatives
- SOCIAL HISTORY: substance use (drugs/alcohol), relational changes or stressors (breakup/divorce, change in living arrangements, job change, or loss), domestic abuse, leisure activities, recent travel, risky sexual behaviors, school/work performance

Ask directed questions about the presence of the following associated symptoms:

- GENERAL APPEARANCE: fever, chills, malaise, pain
- HEAD, EYES, EARS, NECK, AND THROAT (HEENT): headache, photophobia, visual disturbance, sore throat, oral lesions
- NECK: swollen glands, stiffness
- CARDIOVASCULAR (CV): chest pain/pressure, palpitations, extremity edema
- RESPIRATORY: dyspnea, wheezing, cough, position of sleep, exercise tolerance
- ABDOMEN: abdominal pain, nausea/vomiting/diarrhea, stool changes or bleeding
- GENITOURINARY (GU): urinary changes, pregnancy, last menstrual period, excessive bleeding
- MUSCULOSKELETAL: any muscle loss/weakness, trauma, myalgias
- SKIN: rashes, color change (pallor, jaundice)
- LYMPH/HEMATOLOGIC: swollen nodes, any new or excessive bleeding or bruising
- NEUROLOGICAL/PSYCHIATRIC: memory loss, sadness, suicidal ideation, anxiety, seizures, loss of consciousness

Medication History: General

- Medical conditions (treated and untreated), surgeries, allergies, current medications, and over-the-counter therapies
- Medications

Medication History: Specific to Complaint

- Medications
- Vitamins

PHYSICAL EXAMINATION
Vital Signs
- Heart rate (HR)
- Respiratory rate (RR)
- Blood pressure (BP)
- Oxygen saturation (SpO$_2$)
- Temperature

General Appearance
- Alert or lethargic
- Grooming

HENT
- Evidence of trauma
- Oral lesions
- Oropharyngeal erythema

Eyes
- Pupils equal, round, and reactive to light and accommodation (PERRLA)
- External ocular movements
- Conjunctival pallor
- Icterus

Neck
- Lymphadenopathy
- Thyroid enlargement or nodules
- Nuchal rigidity
- Jugular vein distension (JVD)
- Bruits

Cardiovascular
- Rhythm
- Murmurs
- Extra heart sounds
- Extremity edema

Lungs
- Respiratory effort
- Cough
- Air entry
- Adventitious sounds
- Accessory muscle use
- Rubs

Abdomen
- Bowel sounds
- Soft/distended
- Masses
- Tenderness
- Organomegaly

Musculoskeletal
- Muscle bulk and tone
- Acute deformity

- Joint swelling
- Gait

Neurology
- Level of consciousness
- Deep tendon reflexes (DTRs)
- Cranial nerves
- Sensory evaluation
- Memory
- Coordination

Skin
- Pallor
- Bruising or rashes
- Injuries
- Diaphoresis

Psychiatric
- Eye contact
- Affect
- Judgment
- Thought content
- Behavior

CASE STUDY
History

Question	Response
When did the fatigue begin?	*About 3 months ago*
Was the onset sudden or gradual?	*It started right after I was sick with fever. I thought I had strep but they said I didn't.*
Is it improving, worsening, stable, or intermittent?	*It is not getting worse, it just won't go away. I may have been a little less tired this week but it is far from normal. Usually I can run circles around everyone else.*
Were there any suspected precipitating events?	*No, nothing happened that I can remember*
Any recent travel?	*I wish. No.*
Have you had any recent or frequent illnesses?	*I seem to be getting a lot of colds this season*
Any recent sore throat?	*I had a really sore throat with the fever but that went away*
What makes it better or worse?	*Once in a while I can squeeze in a nap*
Are there any associated symptoms?	*No, I'm just tired all the time. I don't feel like exercising and I've gained a few pounds.*
How has it affected your activities of daily living?	*I had to drop an evening class I was taking because I couldn't keep up. The kids always want to play and I just sit on the couch. And our house is a mess.*

Question	Response
What medications are you taking?	*None, just vitamin C and echinacea*
Do you have/have you had any medical conditions?	*I had a thyroid problem when I was pregnant but it got better.*
Are there any medical problems in your family?	*My mother has some sort of thyroid problem that made her gain a lot of weight. My great grandfather had cancer, I don't know what kind.*
How often do you drink alcohol?	*About a glass of red wine a week*
Do you use any substances?	*No I never have. And I don't smoke.*
Have you had any recent stressors?	*Just the night class I was taking. I dropped that. Plus I'm a single mom so it's kinda crazy all the time.*
Do you have any pain or weakness?	*Not really. I get achy when I have a cold but I'm fine right now. No weakness.*
Any severe headaches?	*No, just my regular migraines once in a while*
Any visual changes?	*I got my eyes checked last month and I'm fine*
Any neck discomfort?	*Oh yeah, I almost forgot! I had lumps back here (indicates posterior cervical chain area) for a long time. . . but I don't feel the lumps today.*
Any chest or heart concerns?	*No*
Any difficulty breathing or lung concerns?	*No*
Does your abdomen hurt?	*No*
Any nausea/vomiting or diarrhea?	*No*
Any bleeding in your stool?	*No*
Any urinary concerns?	*No*
Is there any chance you are pregnant?	*No, I tested last week but then my period came the next day*
Do you bleed excessively with your periods?	*The first 2 days I have to change tampons every few hours, then I hardly bleed at all for the next 3 days*
Describe your sleep patterns.	*I want to get to bed just after the kids get to sleep but I have a boyfriend and there is so much to do that often I stay up until 1 a.m. Though I haven't done that so much since dropping my class, but I still have trouble getting to sleep sometimes—my mind races with all I have to do, and sometimes I just get up and do it because I'm not sleepy. I sleep about 6 or 7 hours a night and try to take naps on Sundays or when the kids are sleeping. And I have to get up to pee at night a few times a week.*

Question	*Response*
Any skin changes or rashes?	*Not that I've noticed*
Do you feel depressed or sad?	*Sometimes. I want to be "Fun Mommy" but I don't even want to get up. But I don't think I'm depressed. Just tired.*
Any other symptoms or concerns?	*No. Just that lump if you can find it.*

Physical Examination Findings

- VITAL SIGNS: temperature 98.4°F (oral), heart rate (HR) 60, respiratory rate (RR) 14, blood pressure (BP) 110/72
- GENERAL APPEARANCE: no acute distress; appears fatigued; neatly dressed
- HEENT: no oropharyngeal erythema, within normal limits (WNL)
- EYES: PERRLA 3+, no conjunctival pallor
- NECK/LYMPH: supple, no lymphadenopathy, euthyroid
- CV: regular rhythm, heart sounds normal
- LUNG: normal effort, clear to auscultation
- ABDOMEN: bowel sounds active all four quadrants, soft, nontender, no masses, or organomegaly
- MUSCULOSKELETAL: normal gait and coordination
- NEURO: alert and appropriate
- SKIN: no pallor, bruising, or rashes; warm and dry
- PSYCH: good eye contact, normal affect, and responses

DIFFERENTIAL DIAGNOSIS

Differential Diagnosis	Sleep Deprivation	Mono-nucleosis	Anemia	Hypo-thyroidism	Cardio-pulmonary disease	Neurologic Disorder	Depression	Infectious Process
Onset	Often gradual, unless a specific instigating event	Onset with fever, sore throat	Abrupt or gradual	Usually gradual	Abrupt or gradual	Often abrupt but may be gradual	Often gradual unless a specific instigating event	Abrupt
Shortness of breath	No	No	Yes if severe	No	Often	No	No	If associated with underlying cause
Fever	No	Often at outset	No	No	No unless infectious	Possible	No	Often
Rash	No	Sometimes, especially if treated with penicillin	Can be associated with underlying cause of anemia	No	No	Can be associate with meningitis	No	Possible, depended on illness
Impaired cognition	Possible	No	If severe (due to hypoxia)	Possible	Possible if hypoxic	Possible	Possible following a traumatic event	Possible if septic

DIAGNOSTIC EXAMINATION

Examination	Procedure Code	Cost	Results	Notes
Complete blood count (CBC)	85025	$60+	May indicate anemia (and possible cause), can help differentiate viral versus bacterial etiology, may indicate malignancy	Add iron studies if indicated
Comprehensive metabolic panel (CMP)	80053	$80+	Can indicate electrolyte imbalance, new onset or poorly controlled diabetes, kidney, or liver disease	
Erythrocyte sedimentation rate (ESR)	85652	$60+	Vague inflammatory marker can indicate need for further evaluation and/or rheumatology referral	
Thyroid-stimulating hormone (TSH)	84436	$55+	Indicates underactive thyroid if elevated	Consider adding thyroid antibodies if indicated

CLINICAL DECISION MAKING

Case Study Analysis

The advanced practice nurse notes the following pertinent positives:

- Sudden onset of fatigue 3 months ago after acute fever and sore throat of several days' duration.
- Fatigue is persistent and has caused her to drop a class and miss out on activities she enjoys with her children.

The following are the pertinent negatives:

- No oropharyngeal erythema, no cervical lymphadenopathy
- She has a negative abdominal exam
- Skin exam is WNL

Differential diagnosis analysis:

- Although a primary differential should include mononucleosis, there are also clues to the possibility of anemia (due to heavy menstrual bleeding), thyroid disease (personal and family history), and sleep deprivation (hectic schedule, small children, insomnia).
- A reasonable approach in this case would be to order a CBC, monospot, and thyroid stimulating hormone (TSH) for review.

- When these are performed, the CBC reveals hematocrit and hemoglobin at the low end of normal and lymphocytosis.
- TSH is within normal limits.
- Monospot is positive.

Diagnosis: *Infectious mononucleosis*

FURTHER READING

Holmes, G. P., Kaplan, J. E., Stewart, J. A., Hunt, B., Pinsky, P. F., & Schonberger, L. B. (1987). A cluster of patients with a chronic mononucleosis-type syndrome. Is Epstein–Barr the cause? *Journal of the American Medical Association, 257*(17), 2297.

FOOT PAIN

Case Presentation: A 30-year-old female reports pain in her left foot for the past 4 weeks.

INTRODUCTION TO COMPLAINT

- 64.8% of foot pain is from calluses/corns
- 29.6% of foot pain is caused by hypertrophic nails
- 21.2% hallux deformities (bunion)
- 15.9% from absent arterial pulses

Forefoot Pain

- Ingrown toenails
- Metatarsalgia
- Interdigital neuromas: Morton neuroma
- Hallux rigidus
- Sesamoiditis
- Bunionette
- Callus
- Corns
- Warts
- Metatarsal stress fracture

Midfoot Pain

- Osteoarthritis
- Midfoot planter fasciitis
- Planter fibromas
- Tarsal tunnel syndrome
- Pes planus
- Pes cavus

Hindfoot Pain

- Planter fasciitis

Posterior Heel Pain

- Achilles tendinitis, Haglund's deformity
- Retrocalcaneal bursitis
- Pre-Achilles bursitis
- Achilles rupture

Planter Heel

- Planter surface planter warts

Other Causes

- Possible compartment syndrome
- Deep vein thrombosis
- Sprain of a ligament
- Other fracture aside from stress fracture
- Ruptured tendon

HISTORY OF COMPLAINT

Symptomatology

Ask about the following characteristics of each symptom using open-ended questions:

- Chronology: onset/duration
- Current situation
- Characteristics of pain on a scale of 0 to 10
- Swelling or bruising

Directed Questions to Ask

- When did the symptoms start?
- Did the pain start suddenly or was it gradual over time?
- What time does the pain occur?
- Is it worse at night when lying down or when you first stand up?
- Are there any precipitating factors?
- Are there any other associated symptoms?
- Have you had a previous diagnosis of similar episodes?
- Have you had previous treatments for foot pain?
- Past surgical history?
- What medications do you take?

Assessment: Cardinal Signs and Symptoms

In addition to the general characteristics outlined above, additional characteristics of specific symptoms should be elicited, as follows:

Feet
- Swelling
- Achilles tendon nodules or tenderness
- Heel tenderness
- Malleolus tenderness
- Tenderness over metatarsophalangeal joints
- Range of motion
- Pedal pulses
- Deep tendon reflexes
- Ankle alignment
- Bruising
- Range of motion (ROM)
- Sensation

Medical History: General

- Medical conditions and surgeries
- Allergies

Medical History: Specific to Complaint

- Recent trauma to foot or ankle

PHYSICAL EXAMINATION

Vital Signs

- Temperature
- Pulse
- Respiration
- SpO$_2$
- Blood pressure (BP)

General Appearance

- Apparent state of health: healthy
- Appearance of comfort or distress: very comfortable
- Color: pink
- Nutritional status: well nourished
- State of hydration: no evidence of dehydration
- Hygiene: no problems noted
- Match between appearance and stated age: looks the stated age
- Difficulty with gait or balance: walks favoring the left foot

Ankle and Foot

- INSPECT: Observe all surfaces of the ankles and feet: left foot no nodules no deficiencies, pink, normal disposition of hair on top of great toe, no deformities of bones; foot has normal alignment. Note any deformities, nodules, swelling, calluses, or corns.
- PALPATE: Palpate anterior aspect of each ankle joint, note any bogginess, swelling, or tenderness, feel the Achilles tendon for nodules and tenderness, palpate the heel for tenderness, palpate the medial and lateral malleolus for tenderness, and palpate the meta-tarsophalangeal for tenderness and compress the forefoot between the thumb and fingers.
- ROM AND MANEUVERS: Assess flexion and extension at the ankle joint; assess the inversion and exertion at the subtalar and transverse tarsal joints.
- ASSOCIATED SYSTEMS FOR ASSESSMENT: a complete assessment should include the nervous system (i.e., deep tendon reflexes)

CASE STUDY

History

Question	Response
When did the pain begin?	*Pain began after she started walking 5 miles a day*
What is your current situation?	*Has had to stop walking due to pain*
What are the characteristics of the pain on a scale of 0 to 10?	*Pain a 5 during the day but 10 when she first puts her foot down in the morning*

Question	Response
Is it accompanied by swelling or bruising?	*No*
When did the symptoms start?	*When I put my foot down on the floor in the morning*
Did the pain start suddenly or was it gradual over time?	*Started suddenly but gradually getting worse*
What time does the pain occur?	*When I am walking or standing*
How does the pain affect your daily activities?	*I can't walk for long*
Have you had a previous diagnosis of similar episodes?	*No*
Have you had previous treatments for your foot pain?	*No*
Past surgical history?	*No*
What medications do you take?	*None*
Have you recently taken levoquin? (r/t tendons rupture in some patients)	*No*
Ask the patient to point to the pain?	*Points to plantar surface anterior heel*
Was there an acute injury or overuse from repetitive use of the body part?	*Just walking*
Is there tenderness, warmth, or redness?	*No*
Is there swelling, stiffness, or decreased range of motion?	*No*
What aggravates or relieves the pain?	*Just walking*
What are the effects of exercise, rest, and treatment?	*Rest helps*
Are there any fever or chills?	*No*
Do you have any history of osteoporosis or inflammatory disorders?	*No*
Do you use alcohol or tobacco?	*No*
Do you have any family history of fracture in a first-degree relative?	*No*
Do you use corticosteroids?	*No*
How much do you weigh?	*117 lbs*

Physical Examination Findings

- VITAL SIGNS: temperature 99.2°F, pulse 102, respiration 22, SpO$_2$ (oxygen saturation) 98%, BP 117/72
- GENERAL APPEARANCE: 17-year-old female, 5'3½", 117 lbs

- FEET: ankle and foot have normal color, landmarks, and alignment; both feet are warm with capillary refill less than 1 second. There is tenderness to palpation along the anterior–medial heel of the left foot. Non tender along the Achilles tendon, tarsals, and metatarsals. Full range of motion of the ankle and foot without pain. Dorsalis pedis pulse is 2+ and equal. Sensation is intact to light touch, sharp, and dull.

DIFFERENTIAL DIAGNOSIS

Differential Diagnosis	Plantar Fasciitis	Stress Fracture	Embolic Arterial Occlusion	Deep Vein Thrombosis	Compartment Syndrome
Forefoot		+			
Midfoot	+				
Heel	+				
Swelling		+		+	+
Tenderness on palpation	+	+			
Cold/pallor			+		

DIAGNOSTIC EXAMINATION

Examination	Procedure Code	Cost	Results
Foot x-ray (two views)	73620	$300	These diseases or medical conditions may be diagnosed by, screened for, or associated with foot x-ray: broken foot, broken toe(s), mass or lump in the foot, ligament or cartilage tear, foreign object, infection of the foot, inflammation of the foot.
Ultrasound leg (Doppler)	93971	$100	A Doppler ultrasound test uses reflected sound waves to see how blood flows through a blood vessel. It helps doctors evaluate blood flow through major arteries and veins, such as those of the arms, legs, and neck.
MRI foot	73723	$1500	MRI is a test that uses a magnetic field and pulses of radio wave energy to make pictures of organs and structures inside the body. In many cases, MRI gives different information about structures in the body than can be seen with an x-ray, ultrasound, or CT scan. MRI also may show problems that cannot be seen with other imaging methods.

(*continued*)

Examination	Procedure Code	Cost	Results
CT scan foot	73700	$1100	CT: A diagnostic x-ray or radiological scan in which cross-sectional images of a part of the body are formed through computerized axial tomography and shown on a computer screen.
Bone scan	78300	$200	A bone scan is a test to help find the cause of your back pain. It can be done to find damage to the bones, find cancer that has spread to the bones, and watch problems, such as infection and trauma to the bones. A bone scan can often find problem days to months earlier than a regular x-ray test.

CLINICAL DECISION MAKING

Case Study Analysis

The pertinent positives are a history of sudden pain when getting out of bed. Pain is located over the anterior–medial heel, which is the area of the plantar fascia and is worse with weight bearing and relieved with rest. Pertinent negatives are the absence of trauma, swelling, or decreased pulses.

> *Diagnosis:* *Plantar fasciitis of the left foot*

FURTHER READING

Seller, R. H. (2007). *Differential diagnosis of common complaints* (5th ed.). Philadelphia, PA: Saunders/ Elsevier.

HAND PAIN AND SWELLING

Case Presentation: *A 30-year-old female reports intermittent pain, stiffness, and swelling of her hands for 2 months.*

INTRODUCTION TO COMPLAINT

Joint pain in the hands that is not associated with trauma falls into three general categories:

- Degenerative arthritis: Osteoarthritis (OA)
- Inflammatory arthritis: Rheumatoid, psoriatic, systemic lupus, gout, undifferentiated arthritis
- Joint infection: Parvovirus B19, Lyme disease, or septic joint

> **Clinical Pearls**
> - Morning stiffness lasting more than 60 minutes indicates an inflammatory process
> - The metacarpal (MCP) joints and wrists are painful in rheumatoid arthritis (RA)
> - Distal interphalangeal (DIP) and proximal interphalangeal (PIP) joints are painful in OA

HISTORY OF COMPLAINT

Symptomatology

Ask about the following characteristics of each symptom using open-ended questions:

- Onset
- Location
- Duration/timing
- Character of the pain
- Intensity of the pain
- Triggering factors
- Alleviating factors
- Associated symptoms
- Effect on daily activities
- Previous similar symptoms
- Previous treatment

Directed Questions to Ask

- Is the onset abrupt or gradual?
- What specific joint or joints are affected?
- How long and is it intermittent or constant?
- Is it an ache, burn, sharp, pain, or pressure?
- On a scale of 0 to 10 how severe is the pain?
- Are you stiff when you wake up in the morning? If yes, for how long?
- How many joints are involved?
  - **Monoarthritis:** Is it in one joint?
  - **Polyarthritis:** Is it four or more joints?
- Where is the joint pain?
- Is the joint pain symmetrical?
- Do you have fever, weight loss, malaise, or fatigue?
- How long have the symptoms been present?
- Do you have any rashes?
- Are there any functional losses?
- Do you have other joints that are bothering you now or have bothered you in the past?

Assessment: Cardinal Signs and Symptoms

The following symptoms are associated with joint pain in the hand.

Symptom	Disorder
Constitutional	
Fever, weight loss, and fatigue	Systemic lupus erythematosus, RA
Head, eyes, ears, neck, throat	
Hair loss	SLE, RA
Eye pain, vision loss	Uveitis, temporal arteritis
Conjunctivitis	Reiter's disease
Periorbital edema with violaceous hue	Dermatomyositis
Dry mouth	Sjrogen's disease
Mouth sores	SLE, Bechet's syndrome
Respiratory	
Shortness of breath, pleuritic pain	SLE
Cardiovascular	
Chest pain, palpitation	SLE and RA

(*continued*)

Symptom	Disorder
Gastrointestinal	
Abdominal pain, nausea, and vomiting; diarrhea	SLE
Gastroenteritis	Reactive arthritis
Genitourinary	
Urethral discharge, urethritis	Reiter's syndrome
Psychiatric	
Personality change	SLE
Neurologic	
Headaches, numbness tingling, seizures	SLE
Skin	
Malar rash, photosensitive rashes	SLE
Slapped cheek	Human parvovirus B19
Annular red plague (*Erythema migrans*)	Lyme disease
Violaceous papules/plaques on hand	Dermatomyositis
Psoriatic plaque, nail pitting	Psoriatic arthritis

Medical History: General

- Active problem, list of past medical problems
- Past surgeries
- Current medications and drug allergies
- Family history of inflammatory arthritis, inflammatory bowel disease, thyroiditis
- Occupation, living situation, exercise, alcohol, nicotine, illicit drugs

Medical History: Specific to Complaint

- Family history of inflammatory arthritis, inflammatory bowel disease, thyroiditis
- Pain with range of motion to hand and wrist
- Inability to hold heavy objects
- Localized swelling

PHYSICAL EXAMINATION
Vital Signs

- Blood pressure (BP)
- SpO$_2$ (oxygen saturation)

General Appearance

Eyes
- Inspect for conjunctivitis or excessive dry eye

Mouth
- Inspect for sores or dry mouth

Heart
- Listen for murmur, rub, or abnormal rhythm

Abdomen
- Palpate for enlarged liver or spleen

Musculoskeletal
- Palpate all joints and note deformity, swelling, redness, heat, or tenderness
  - OA tends to have bony enlargement of the DIP and PIP joints
  - RA tends to have a spongy texture (synovial effusion) over the joints
  - Gout is too tender to touch
  - Psoriatic arthritis occurs in the DIP joints and may appear as a "sausage digit" with swelling of the tendon sheath of the finger; nail pitting may be observed

Skin
- Observe the skin for rashes, especially in sun-exposed areas of the face

CASE STUDY
History

Question	Response
Was the onset of your joint pain sudden or gradual?	*Gradual, over days*
Can you show me what joints are bothering you?	*[Points to all metacarpals]*
How long have you had the joint pain?	*About 2 months*
Is it constant or intermittent?	*It started coming and going and now it is constant*
Have you had it before?	*Yes, it was there a month ago*
Does anything seem to trigger it?	*No, I have felt fine till this*
Does anything make it better?	*Ibuprofen helps a bit*
Can you describe how the pain feels?	*It is a constant ache*
On a scale of 0 to 10 how severe is the pain?	*Probably 5 or 6*
Do you have swelling or redness with the pain?	*Yes, especially in the morning*
Are your hands stiff?	*Yes, all day, so stiff*
Has it affected your daily activities?	*Yes, I it is hard to button things*
Has anyone ever had this in your family?	*Yes, my mom had RA*

Question	Response
Do you have any fevers, weight loss of fatigue	*No, the pain is tiring*
Do you have any hair loss or rashes	*Not that I've noticed*
Do any other joints hurt you	*Right now, just my hands*

Physical Examination Findings

- VITAL SIGNS: temperature 98.8°F, HR 64, respiratory rate 16, BP 90/60, height 5′2″, weight 110 lbs
- GENERAL APPEARANCE: healthy-appearing female in no acute pain
- EYES: no injection, pupils equal, round, and reactive to light and accommodation (PERRLA)
- NARES: patent, no discharge
- MOUTH: mucus membranes moist, no oral lesions or dental caries
- NECK: thyroid is not palpable, no adenopathy
- HEART: normal S2 and S2 without murmur gallop or rub
- ABDOMEN: soft, nontender without mass or organomegaly

Hands
- INSPECTION: hands reveal mild swelling of the MCP and PIP joints; faint redness
- PALPATION: notable for effusion of the joints with moderate tenderness and warmth
- RANGE OF MOTION: limited in flexion of the MCP and PIP joints; normal extension
- STRENGTH: hand grip is 4/5 bilaterally

Wrist
- INSPECTION: moderate swelling of the joints bilaterally, no redness
- PALPATION: notable for effusion of the wrists, moderate tenderness
- RANGE OF MOTION: limited flexion, normal extension
- STRENGTH: 4/5 flexion and extension, ulnar and radial deviation
- JOINT SURVEY: sterno-clavicular (SC), acromio-clavicular (AC) shoulder, elbow, hip, knee, ankle, feet no evidence of joint swelling, redness, tenderness, decreased range of motion or limitations in strength

Neurovascular
- PULSES: brachial, dorsalis pedis, and radial pulse 2+ and equal
- SENSATION: intact to light touch, sharp distal extremities

DIFFERENTIAL DIAGNOSIS

Disease	Risk Factors	Common Symptoms	Common Signs	Other	Diagnostic Test
Rheumatoid	F:M 3:1 Family history Common	Gradual onset of symmetric pain in small joints of hands and feet with prolonged am stiffness	Joint effusions, tenderness restricted motion MCP, wrists	Fatigue, fever weight loss	+ RF _+ anti-CCP, high ESR and CRP

(continued)

Disease	Risk Factors	Common Symptoms	Common Signs	Other	Diagnostic Test
Systemic lupus	F:M 9:1, African American three times greater, age 13 to 40, family history	Gradual onset of symmetric arthritis, morning stiffness with systemic symptoms	Joint effusion, tenderness, restricted motion MCP, wrists, malar rash, pleuritis, pericarditis	Fatigue, photosensitive skin rash, oral ulcerations, psychiatric illness, parasthesia	+ antinuclear antibody ANA antidouble stranded DNA, anti-Smith antibody, anemia, proteinuria
Human Parvovirus	Exposed to small children	Gradual onset of symmetrical joint pain in MCP, PIP < 6 weeks	Small joints of hands, wrists, and feet, restricted motion	Slapped-cheek rash	Immunoglobulin (Ig) M antibodies to human parvovirus B19 +
Fibromyalgia	F:M 9:1 age 30 to 50, genetic, environmental	Muscle pain, aching, fatigue, stiffness, poor sleep	No joint swelling or tenderness, muscle tenderness, + trigger points	Fatigue is common but no fever or rash	Clinical diagnosis + tender points 11/18

CCP, citrullinated peptide; CRP, C-reactive protein; ESR, erythrocyte sedimentation rate; MCP, metacarpal; RF, rheumatoid factor.

DIAGNOSTIC EXAMINATION

Examinations	Procedure Code	Cost	Indications and Interpretation
X-ray or plain film	73130	$250	Early in inflammatory joint disease and arthritis, radiographic findings are subtle or absent. In RA you may see erosions, deformities, and demineralization of bone. Good to get a baseline for future reference of joint changes.
Rheumatoid factor	86430	$180	Positive in 85% of patients with RA, nonspecific, can be elevated in other inflammatory on infectious processes
Anti-citrullinated protein antibody	86200	$275	Specific to RA; present in 50% to 80% of patients
Antinuclear antibodies	86038	$180	+ ANA and specific nuclear antibodies are present in RA and SLE
C-reactive protein	86140	$150	Nonspecific but elevated in most inflammatory arthritis

Examinations	Procedure Code	Cost	Indications and Interpretation
Erythrocyte sedimentation rate	85652	$75	Nonspecific but elevated in most inflammatory arthritis, slower to rise and lower than CRP
Complete blood count	85025	$75	Inflammatory arthritis is associated with anemia of chronic disease; septic joint will have elevated white blood count
Basic metabolic panel	80048	$119	Systemic inflammatory arthritis is associated with nephritis or renal failure
Urinalysis	81003	$25	Establishes presence or absence of proteinuria or red cell cast + SLE
Liver enzymes and function	83516	$120	Usually negative unless autoimmune hepatitis; establish baseline for future drug treatment
Lyme titer Western blot	86618	$180	In endemic areas especially in the presence of erythema migrans
Parvovirus B19 antibodies IgM and IgG	83520	$200	If polyarthritis is less than 6-week duration can rule out parvovirus; if positive for IGM antibody, recent infection is present

IgG, immunoglobulin G; IgM, immunoglobulin M.

The 2010 American College of Rheumatology Classification for Rheumatoid Arthritis

Who should be tested?
1. Patients with at least one joint with definite synovitis on examination
2. Patients with synovitis not explained by any other disease

Joint Involvement	Score
One joint	0
Two to 10 joints	1
One to three small joints	2
Four to 10 small joints	3
Greater than 10 joints	4

(continued)

Joint Involvement	Score
Serology	
Negative rheumatoid factor (RF) and CCP-antibody	0
Low-positive RF or low-positive CCP-antibody	2
High-positive RF or high-positive CCP-antibody	3
Acute-phase reactants	
Normal CRP and normal ESR	0
Abnormal CRP or normal ESR	1
Duration of symptoms	
< 6 weeks	0
> 6 weeks	1

A score of 6 out of 10 indicates the patient has RA.

CLINICAL DECISION MAKING

Case Study Analysis

The advanced practice nurse (APN) notes that the patient's test results are as follows:

- Normal complete blood count, complete metabolic panel
- Elevated CRP and ESR
- Negative rheumatoid factor
- Negative antinuclear antibody
- Elevated CCP antibody
- X-rays show joint effusions of the MCP and PIPs, but no erosions

The APN has evaluated the 30-year-old woman who presents with recurrent episodes of symmetric pain and swelling in MCP joints and wrists for 2 months. Her history is significant for a family history of RA in her mother. She does not have systemic symptoms of fevers, weight loss, fatigue, or rashes, which could indicate possible systemic lupus. Her symptoms have been present for over 6 weeks making the diagnosis of human parvovirus unlikely. Her examination reveals symmetric joint pain and effusions of the MCP and wrists, which is a common finding in rheumatoid arthritis. She meets the criteria for diagnostic testing and her laboratory test confirms the presence of the CCP-antibody, elevated CRP and ESR. Her x-rays do not reveal an erosive arthritis, but this is common in early stage of disease.

Diagnosis: *Diagnosis is rheumatoid arthritis*

FURTHER READING

Ferri, F. F. (2011). *Ferri's clinical advisor*. St. Louis, MO: Elsevier Mosby.

Klippel, J. H., Weyand, C. M, Crofford, L. J., & Stone, J. H. (2001). *Primer on the rheumatic diseases* (12th ed.). Atlanta, GA: Arthritis Foundation.

Mies Reichi, A., & Francis, M. L. (2003). Diagnostic approach to polyarticular joint pain. *American Family Physician, 68*(6), 1151–1160.

Wasserman, A. M. (2011). Diagnosis and management of rheumatoid arthritis. *American Family Physician, 84*(11), 1245–1252.

HEADACHE

Case Presentation: A 25-year-old Hispanic female presents to your clinic with a headache.

INTRODUCTION TO COMPLAINT

This is one of the most complicated presenting complaints that a nurse practitioner commonly treats. Over 90% of headaches are benign, and most commonly are either migraine or tension headaches. However, there are several quite serious etiologies that must first be ruled out.

Common Headache Without Fever

Migraines are familial and most often unilateral. Photophobia, nausea, and vomiting are common presenting symptoms. Tension headaches are often bilateral and are accompanied by muscular neck and shoulder pain. Cluster headaches are more common in men and are sharp and of short duration. They occur several times in a short time period. Often they are accompanied by unilateral rhinitis and tearing.

Other Headaches Without Fever to Consider

Sinusitis, rhinosinusitis, space-occupying lesions, cancer, hypertension (HTN), posttraumatic stress, vessel abnormalities, and bleeding within the brain need to be assessed.

Headache With Fever

If a fever is present, the most common reason is infectious meningitis. This is accompanied by meningeal signs of pain to the neck that increase when the head is flexed and the knees are bent (Bruzinski and Kernig signs). It is also possible to have a headache as a reaction to a systemic disease or a brain abscess.

Other

A few rare etiologies for headache are familial hemiplegic migraine, pituitary apoplexy, and malignancy of the central nervous system (CNS).

Triggers

Migraines have specific triggers that, when avoided, can prevent onset. These are often tension, lack of sleep, red wine, avocados, and aged cheese, but can be anything. In women, the menstrual cycle can be a trigger.

HISTORY OF COMPLAINT

Symptomatology

Ask about the following characteristics of each symptom using open-ended questions:

- Onset (sudden or gradual) of current headache and age of onset of headaches
- Location
- Duration, frequency, intensity of each episode
- Character (aching, sharp, dull, burning)
- Associated symptoms (presence or absence of aura, fever, rhinitis)
- Radiation
- Timing (morning, evening, after exercise or stress)
- Severity
- Precipitating and aggravating factors
- Relieving factors
- Effects on daily activities
- Previous diagnosis of similar episodes
- Previous treatments
- Efficacy of previous treatments
- Family history of similar episodes
- History of past workup (computed tomography [CT], MRI)

Directed Questions to Ask

- Was the onset sudden (thunderclap) or gradual?
- Do you have fever? (intracranial, systemic, local infection)
- Is this the first or worst headache of your life? (intracranial hemorrhage, CNS abnormality)
- New headache (HA) under 5 or over 50?
- Worsening pattern? (mass, subdural hemorrhage [SDH], overuse)
- Focal neurologic signs/symptoms other than typical visual or sensory aura? (mass, arterial/ventricular malformation [AVM], collagen vascular diagnosis)
- Rapid onset with strenuous activity, especially if preceded by trauma? (carotid artery dissection or intracranial hemorrhage)
- History of cancer? (metastasis)
- History of Lyme disease? (meningoencephalitis)
- HIV+? (opportunistic infection or tumor)
- Pregnant or postpartum? (cortical vein or venous sinus thrombosis, carotid dissection, pituitary ipoplexy)

Assessment: Cardinal Signs and Symptoms

In addition to the general characteristics outlined above, additional characteristics of specific symptoms should be elicited, as follows:

Head, Eyes, Ears, Nose, Throat (HEENT)
- Eye tearing
- Vision changes
- Rhinitis, allergies, recent upper respiratory illness
- Pain over sinuses
- Ear pain

Neck

- Pain to the musculature and to shoulders
- Increased pain when flexing the head or bending the knees

Other Associated Symptoms

- Fever
- Nausea, vomiting, flashing lights, aura, or prodrome
- Change in mental status, personality, or level of consciousness
- High blood pressure (BP)

Medical History: General

- Medical conditions and surgeries
- Allergies (seasonal as well as others)
- Herbal preparations and traditional therapies

Medical History: Specific to Complaint

- History of sinusitis
- Seasonal allergies
- Past headaches and effective treatments
- Recent trauma (can be as long as 3 months prior to onset of HA)
- History of cancer
- Exposure to meningitis
- History of meningococcal vaccine

PHYSICAL EXAMINATION

Vital Signs

- BP (very high with pheochromocytoma)
- Heart rate (HR)
- Temperature

General Appearance

- Appearance of comfort or distress
- Wearing dark glasses or in darkened room

HEENT

- SCALP/TEMPLES: palpate for areas of tenderness (trauma/temporal arteritis over temples in middle aged women)
- EYES: clear sclera, fundoscopy looking for papilledema (increased intracranial pressure), presence of tearing (cluster); visual field defects (lesion of the optic pathway, pituitary mass), impaired vision or seeing "holes" around a light (glaucoma, subacute angle closure glaucoma); blurred vision when bending forward that improves with sitting up (elevated intracranial pressure [ICP]); blurred vision relieved with recumbancy and exacerbated with upright posture (low ICP); complete sudden loss of vision unilaterally (optic neuritis)
- EARS: tympanic membranes grey with light reflex, clear canals (acute otitis media)
- NARES: edema, discharge (rhinosinusitis)
- SINUS CAVITIES: tenderness with tapping, increase in pain with forward flexion (sinusitis)
- Flex neck (Brudzinski) assessing for increased headache pain that causes flexion of the knees for relief (meningitis, subarachnoid hemorrhage [SAH], encephalitis)

- NUCHAL RIGIDITY: inability to flex neck (meningitis)
- Palpate trapezius and sterno-cleido-mastoid (SCM) muscles and cervical vertebrae (tension)
- Carotid bruits (heard on the opposite side as the arterio-venous malformation [AVM])

Abdomen
- Assess for tenderness (if nausea/vomiting present)

Neurologic
- PERRLA (pupils equal, round, and reactive to light and accommodation); EOMs (extraocular movements) intact and without pain to movement
- Cranial nerves
- Equal strength to head, upper extremity (UE), and lower extremity (LE)
- Sensation equal bilaterally to face, UE, and LE
- DTRs (deep tendon reflexes) 2+, equal bilaterally (cerebellar abnormalities)
- FUNCTIONAL NEUROLOGIC EXAMINATION: Get up from seated position without support, walk on tiptoes and heels, tandem gait. Cerebellar: Romberg, pronator drift. Finger to nose, rapid alternating fingers

CASE STUDY

History

Question	Response
Have you had this before?	Yes, it started when I was 15, with menses
Is this headache similar to past ones?	Yes, it is just the same
How often do you have them?	Usually once a month for about 3 days
What helps?	Usually rest, ibuprofen, and sleep, but it is annoying to have to sleep all day
Have you tried any medicine?	No
Does anyone else have this?	Yes, my mom. She has a shot that helps.
Where does it hurt?	Right temporal
Does your neck hurt?	No
Have you noticed a change to vision, your mental status, or speech?	No
Did it start gradually?	Yes, it was not that bad at first, then increased
What is the quality and severity?	It is an 8 to 10 right now and stabbing and throbbing
Do you have trouble with light, sound?	Yes, I have to wear dark glasses, sound is okay
Any nausea or vomiting?	No vomiting, but I am very nauseous
Have you been able to drink water?	Not as much as I should. I am so nauseous.
Have you had a fever? Neck pain?	No. No.
Have you had any injury to your head?	No

Question	Response
Have you had vision change, dizziness?	*No*
Any new stressors?	*No, I go to school, but it's always stressful*
Chronic nasal stuffiness or sinusitis?	*Seasonal allergies, but not now*
Any pain with urination, flank pain?	*No*
What do you think brought this one on?	*Well, it seems to be related to starting my period. Mine is due. It usually happens just before my period starts. I also notice red wine and I did drink a glass the night before it started. I read about avocados and cheese, but I don't notice anything with them.*
Do you use any drugs? Smoke?	*No*
Have you ever been pregnant?	*No*
What is your menstrual cycle?	*28 days, regular, with 3 days of flow*
What other health problems do you have?	*Seasonal allergies and headaches*
Surgery?	*No*
What medications do you take?	*Claritin and ibuprofen as needed, Ortho Tri-Cyclen Lo*
Allergies to medicine?	*No*
Tell me about your family history?	*My mom has migraines and fibromyalgia; my dad has kidney stones*
FMH of AVM, tumors, cancer, hypertension, myocardial infarction, cerebrovascular accident?	*No*

Physical Examination Findings

- VITAL SIGNS: 98.6°F; respiratory rate (RR) 16; heart rate (HR) 86, regular; blood pressure (BP) 100/60
- GENERAL APPEARANCE: well-developed, healthy appearing female wearing dark glasses in a dim room; she is not smiling, but is answering appropriately.
- EYES: no injection, anicteric, PERRLA, EOMs intact, without pain to movement; normal vision
- NOSE: nares are patent; no edema or exudate of turbinates
- Tympanic membranes grey with light reflex, canals clear
- OROPHARYNX: no lesions, edema, exudates, or erythema; good dentition
- NECK: supple, full range of motion (FROM) without pain to palpation over the cervical vertebrae or the trapezius, SCM muscles; no increase in pain with neck flexion
- No carotid bruits
- CHEST: lungs are clear in all fields; heart S1 S2 no murmur, gallop, or rub
- ABDOMEN: soft, nontender without mass or organomegaly
- SKIN: no rashes
- EXTREMITIES: equal strength bilaterally to head, UE, and LE; no edema
- NEUROLOGIC: Cranial nerves II to XII intact; sensation intact, DTRs 2+ throughout
- Functional neurological examination is normal

DIFFERENTIAL DIAGNOSIS

Differential Diagnosis	Common Symptoms	Signs
Migraines	Unilateral, nausea and vomiting (N/V), photophobia	Normal neurological examination, appears uncomfortable, wearing sunglasses
Tension	Entire head or band, often with neck/shoulders, stressors	Neck pain, normal neurology
Cluster	Unilateral, male, short duration Occurs in clusters	Unilateral rhinitis, tearing
Sinusitis	Rhinitis, frontal pressure	Nare edema, sinus cavities tender to palpation (TTP)
Meningitis	Nuchal rigidity, photophobia Headache	Appears ill, Kernig/Bruzinski +
Temporal arteritis	> 55, HA, fatigue, malaise, night sweats	Tender to temples
Overuse HA	Daily headache, using meds daily	Depends on type of HA
Brain tumor	New/worse HA, vision change	Neurological changes
Post-traumatic	Pain at site of injury, head injury	Neurological changes
Systemic reaction	fever, associated ill symptoms	Relieves with lower temperature

DIAGNOSTIC EXAMINATION

Examination	Procedure Code	Cost	Results
Fundoscopy	NA	Part of examination	If you are seeing engorgement of the veins without pulsation, hemorrhages near the optic disc, blurring of the optic margins, or elevation of the optic disc, this is a sign of papilledema, which is indicative of increased intracranial pressure. You may also see "Paton's lines," which are radial retinal lines that originate at the optic disc and radiate outward
CBC	85025	$32 to $75	You will see an elevated white blood count (WBC) in systemic infection
Lumbar puncture (LP): concern for SAH with a negative CT OR suspected infection	62270	$190 to $350	This is not done in a clinic; the patient would be sent to the emergency department or scheduled for interventional radiology if nonemergent; the cerebral spinal fluid (CSF) would not be clear and there would be bacteria, crystals, white blood cells in the fluid; this can be further tested for bacteria or viruses

(*continued*)

Examination	Procedure Code	Cost	Results
CT: trauma with loss of consciousness or vomiting OR nonacute HA with abnormal neurological examination OR for reassurance of the patient (particularly if FMH of tumor)	70450	$1290 to $3000	You could see a large mass or a hematoma signifying an area of bleeding within the brain structure; the type of bleed is determined by the location: SAH versus SDH
MRI/MRA (magnetic resonance arteriogram): to see masses not seen on CT or for vessel damage FMH of AVM	70553 or 70544	$4097 $2585	You could see an AVM or a mass not seen on CT or an aneurysm

CLINICAL DECISION MAKING

It is important to rule out all the danger signs first. Often this can be done with a thorough history. A neurological examination is essential. If this is abnormal, the patient needs to be referred for imaging and to a neurologist, which is best handled in the emergency department. If there are no danger signs and no neurological changes on the examination, you can be reassured that this is a benign headache.

Case Study Analysis

The advance practice nurse (APN) performs the assessment and physical examination on the patient and finds the following: 25-year-old woman with a HA of 3 days that is similar to her history of HAs. She endorses photophobia and nausea. It is an 8 to 10 with throbbing and stabbing pain. There is a correlation with her menses, which is due and with red wine. Denies red flags of trauma, fever, vomiting, vision changes, neurological changes.

She fits the International Headache Society criteria for diagnosis of migraine: at least five attacks lasting 4 to 72 hours, unilateral, pulsating, moderate to severe intensity, causing avoidance of routine activity, associated with nausea and photophobia.

Diagnosis: *Migraine headache*

HEARTBURN

Case Presentation: A 40-year-old Mexican American male presents with "my stomach hurts after I eat."

INTRODUCTION TO COMPLAINT

Heartburn (pyrosis) is a common complaint in primary care practice. It is described as a burning sensation in the central chest, typically after eating:

- The majority of heartburn cases are benign and related to one of three types of problems:
  - Mucosal irritation
    - Gastroesophageal reflux
    - Peptic ulcer disease (PUD)
    - Intermittent reflux due to obesity, large meals, fatty foods, caffeine, or alcohol
  - *Helicobacter pylori* infection
  - Nonulcer dyspepsia
- Other causes of heartburn-like symptoms are:
  - Mechanical: pregnancy, hiatal hernia, esophogeal strictures
  - Iatrogenic: large pill volume, medication induced, radiation induced
  - Motility: lower esophogeal hypotension, esophageal dysmotility
  - Inflammatory: eosinophilic esophagitis, scleroderma, sarcoidosis
  - Vascular: angina, intestinal ischemia
  - Cancerous: esophageal, gastric or duodenal cancers, gastrinoma
- The VBAD mnemonic (very bad) reminds you of the most alarming features to look for:
  - Vomiting
  - Bleeding: anemia
  - Abdominal mass
  - Dysphagia (pain when swallowing—especially with solids or if worsening)
- Other alarming features by body system include:
  - General: evolving—progressive symptoms, weight loss, age > 45 years
  - Abdominal: jaundice, rigid abdomen, pulsatile abdomen
  - Stool—emesis: hematochezia, melena, hematemesis, coffee-ground emesis
  - Pain: acute onset, severe quantity, ripping, tearing quality

HISTORY OF COMPLAINT

Symptomatology

A systematic process for obtaining a history will support accurate diagnosis and testing.

Ask the about the following characteristics of each symptom using open-ended questions:

- Provocative and palliative factors
- Quantity and quality of pain or symptoms

- Region and radiation of pain or symptoms
- Symptoms associated with the chief complaint
- Time course and therapies tried
- Patient understanding of the symptom's cause and its impact on his or her life

Directed Questions to Ask

- When did your pain begin? *or* When did you *first* have this pain?
- What makes your pain worse? *and* What makes it better?
- What words describe how your pain feels?
- If 0 is no pain and 10 is the worst pain you can imagine, what number is your pain?
- Where is your pain located; can you point to it?
- Do you also feel pain in other places at the same time—like your belly, back, or chest?
- Have you noticed any other new symptoms since your belly pain began?
- When the pain comes, how long does it last—minutes, hours, or days?
- After you eat, how long does it take before the pain starts?
- Have you tried anything to help the pain (suggest things like herbs, over-the-counter (OTC) drugs, prescriptions)?
- What do you think is causing the pain? How has it affected your day-to-day life?

Assessment: Cardinal Signs and Symptoms

Four systems are assessed: (a) general, (b) abdominal (involved), (c) head/eye/ear/neck/throat (HEENT) or pulmonary (above), and (d) genitourinary (GU) or musculoskeletal–spine (below)

- General: nausea, vomiting, diarrhea, weight loss, difficulty swallowing
- Above (pulmonary): shortness of breath, coughing, chest pain
- Involved (abdominal): abdominal changes (rigid or pulsatile), stool changes (bright red blood or thick-black-tarry stools), vomiting (hematemesis or coffee emesis)
- Below (GU): urine changes (dark color, bloody, painful)

Medical History: General

- Good health with no significant history
- Surgical: abdominal injury or surgery
- Medications: use of calcium channel blockers (CCBs), inhalers, tricyclics, iron, potassium, tetracycline
- Nutrition: large-volume meals
  - High-fat foods (including fast foods, oils, butter, red meats)
  - Acidic liquids (soda, citrus juices)
  - Acidic foods: liquids (citrus, tomato)
  - Other foods (spices, chocolates, peppermint, garlic)
- Substances: alcohol, tobacco, recreational drugs (cocaine, heroin, marijuana)

Medical History: Specific to Complaint

- Stomach disorders (like reflux, ulcers, or cancer)
- Intestinal disorders (like IBS, IBD, or colitis)
- Liver–gallbladder disorders (like hepatitis, cirrhosis, or gallstones)

- Pancreatic disorders (like pancreatitis or diabetes)
- Lung disorders (like emphysema, asthma, or TB)
- Renal and genital disorders (like renal failure, kidney stones)
- Patient could not recall eating or drinking anything that caused this complaint

PHYSICAL EXAMINATION

The physical examination serves to exclude alarming pathologies but is not very useful for determining the exact cause of heartburn. A systematic examination can include:

Vital Signs

- Blood pressure (BP)
- Pulse
- Temperature

General Appearance

- Anthropometry: body mass index (BMI), height, weight, abdominal girth

Involved

Abdominal
- Contour
- Bowel sounds: four quadrants
- Tenderness to palpation and location of tenderness
- Spleen–liver size by palpation and percussion
- Abdominal masses
- Fluid shift
- Tests and signs: McBurney's Blumberg, McMurphy, Markle, Cullen, Grey-Turner

Above

Pulmonary–Chest
- Auscultation of anterior–posterior–lateral fields
- Egophany

Cardiovascular
- Auscultation of S1, S2 for rate, rhythm, murmurs, rubs, gallops
- Abdominal bruits or pulsations
- EKG for unexplained chest pain only

Below

Musculoskeletal
- Sternum–rib joint stability and tenderness
- Lumbar–thoracic range of motion, joint stability, and deformities

HEENT (Optional and Mostly for Detecting Atypical Reflux Sequelae)

- Dentition: presence–absence, coloration, caries, erosions, repairs
- Oral mucosal: coloration, lesions
- Oropharynx: tonsilar size, erythema, edema

CASE STUDY
History

Question	Response
What brings you in today?	*I have pain in my stomach—it is frustrating!*
Tell me about your pain.	*It hurts badly after I eat*
When did your pain begin?	*Oh, I don't know. Maybe 6 months ago.*
What makes your pain worse?	*It happens mostly after lunch and dinner. Breakfast doesn't seem to bother it.*
Does any food or drink make it worse?	*It is really mostly when I have more than 8 tortillas at once or carne asada (grilled beef)*
What makes your pain better?	*I don't really know*
What word describes your pain?	*It is like a fire in my chest and a deep ache in my belly after I eat*
What number would you give your pain?	*3*
Show me where your pain is.	*[Places hand on epigastrium and sternum]*
When you have pain in your belly, do you feel pain anywhere else—like your abdomen, back, chest, or throat?	*Yes—in the center of my chest*
Are there any other symptoms you have noticed since your belly pain began?	*No*
How long does the pain last?	*Well, I guess it usually stays for about 2 hours or so after I eat*
Have you tried anything like vitamins, herbs, prescriptions, or over-the-counter medicines to help the pain?	*Yes; Maalox seems to help it some and ibuprofen seems to make it better for a bit*
What do you think is causing the pain?	*I don't know. That is why I came to see you.*

Physical Examination Findings

- VITAL SIGNS: 98.7°F; heart rate (HR) 86, regular; respiratory rate (RR) 16; blood pressure (BP) 130/74; height 74"; weight 334 lbs; body mass index (BMI) 42.9
- GENERAL APPEARANCE: no acute distress, elevated BMI
- PULMONARY: clear to auscultation anteriorly, posteriorly, and laterally without wheezes, rhonchi, or rales; no egpohany; no retractions
- CARDIOVASCULAR: S1 and S2 within normal limits; no murmurs, rubs, or gallops; no S3 or S4; no abdominal bruits or palpable abdominal pulsations
- ABDOMINAL: bowels sounds present ×4 quadrants, protrubent abdomen with striae; mild tenderness to palpation in epigastrium and along medial costal margins bilaterally no hepatosplenomegaly appreciated by palpation or percussion but examination limited by abdominal girth of 154 cm (at umbilicus); negative Blumberg, Murphy's, McBurney's, Markle, Grey–Turner, and Cullen signs; no fluid shift
- MUSCULOSKELETAL: sternum–rib joints stable and no tenderness to palpation

DIFFERENTIAL DIAGNOSIS

The table summarizes symptoms of intermittent reflux, gastroesophageal disease (GERD), peptic ulcer disease (PUD), and nonulcer dyspepsia. Symptoms alone can suggest possible causes of heartburn.

Symptoms	GERD	PUD	Nonulcer Dyspepsia	Intermittent Reflux
30- to 60-minute postprandial onset	Common	If gastric	Common	Common
Steady discomfort for 30 to 120 minutes	Common	Common	Possible	Common
Food intake triggers pain	Common	If gastric	Common	Common
Retrosternal burning quality	Common	Uncommon	Uncommon	Common
Reflux (stomach contents in mouth or throat)	Common	–	–	Possible
Specific food triggers (fatty, spicy, acidic)	Common	Common	–	Common
Liquid triggers (sodas, alcohol, caffeine)	Common	Common	–	Common
Nonsteroidal anti-inflammatory drugs (NSAIDs) trigger	Common	Common	–	Common
Epigastric pain	Common	Common	Common	Uncommon
Supine position triggers	Common	–	–	Common
Bitter taste in mouth	Common	–	–	Common
Epigastric burning	Uncommon	Common	Common	Common
Nocturnal pain awakens from sleep	Uncommon	If duodenal	–	–
Nausea: mild and intermittent	Uncommon	Uncommon	Common	–
Belching, postprandial	Uncommon	Common	Common	–
Bloating	Uncommon	Common	Common	–
Chronic cough	Uncommon	–	–	–
Laryngitis (hoarseness)	Uncommon	–	–	Uncommon

(*continued*)

Symptoms	GERD	PUD	Nonulcer Dyspepsia	Intermittent Reflux
Halitosis (bad breath)	Uncommon	–	–	–
Throat clearing	Uncommon	–	–	–
Hypersalivation (water brash)	Rare	–	–	–
Globus (throat fullness despite swallow)	Rare	–	–	–
Dental erosions	Rare	–	–	–
Epigastric "fullness" (postprandial)	Rare	Uncommon	Common	Uncommon
Vomiting: mild and intermittent	Rare	Uncommon	–	–
"Gnawing," "hunger-like," or "achy" quality	–	Common	–	Uncommon
2- to 5-hour postprandial onset	–	If duodenal	–	Uncommon
Food relieves pain	–	If duodenal	–	–
Early satiety	–	Common	Common	Uncommon
Psychiatric comorbidity	–	Rare	Common	–
Relapse–remitting pain pattern	–	–	Common	Common

DIAGNOSTIC EXAMINATION

- Initiate lifestyle modification for heartburn trigger reduction and/or
- Conduct a "PPI test"; this is an empiric GERD therapy with a high-dose proton pump inhibitor (PPI) at least 30 to 60 minutes before meals (AC) twice daily (BID)
  - A "PPI test" is positive and suggests GERD if symptoms resolve within 4 weeks
  - Common agents are: Omeprazole 20 mg or Lansoprazole 30 mg
  - Diagnostic testing for heartburn is typically reserved for patients with:
    - Failed PPI test
    - Alarm symptoms
    - Recurrence of symptoms within 3 months after successful suppression using a PPI
    - History clearly suggestive of a non-GERD pathology (e.g., *H. pylori* or hiatal hernia)

Examination	Procedure Code	Cost	Results
Stool antigen, *H. pylori* or *H. pylori* urea breath test	87338	$25	A positive result would indicate active infection A negative result would indicate no active infection
Red blood cell (RBC) count and indices (hemoglobin [Hgb], hematocrit [Hct], and mean corpuscular volume [MCV] are part of a complete blood count)	85027	$20	RBC count = 4.50 Hgb = 13.5 Hct = 40.5 MCV = 90.0 All of the patient's studies were within normal limits. Anemia is present if the total number of RBCs, Hgb, and/or Hct is below the normal range for the patient's age and sex. The MCV cutoffs for RBC size in adults are: < 80: Microcytic (small cells) 80 to 100: Normocytic (normal sized cells) > 100: Macrocytic (large cells) However, a normocytic or microcytic anemia, if present, could suggest an active gastrointestinal bleed
Endoscopy	43200	$1000	Referral to gastroenterology for refractory symptoms

CLINICAL DECISION MAKING

Case Study Analysis

The clinician's examination does not identify a focal cause of the patient's heartburn or any alarming features (such as hypotension, tachycardia, or abdominal masses). However, the patient's positive *H. pylori* stool antigen indicates an active infection that likely caused PUD. His postprandial, gnawing epigastric pain is consistent with PUD.

> **Diagnosis:** *Peptic ulcer disease secondary to* H. pylori *infection*

- Additional PUD risks include heavy alcohol use, NSAID use, and central adiposity
- The patient's normal RBC indices suggest the ulcer is not a cause of significant blood loss
- Causes of heartburn are not mutually exclusive and can often overlap; however, key symptoms inhibit prostaglandins that protect the mucosal wall from stomach acidity
- Alcohol intake can damage the mucosa directly due to acidity
- Central adiposity may compress the esophageal sphincter and promote reflux

FURTHER READING

Barter, C., & Dunne, L. (2011). Abdominal pain. In J. E. South-Paul, S. C. Matheny, & E. L. Lewis (Eds.), *Current diagnosis and treatment in family medicine* (3rd ed., pp. 319–336). New York, NY: McGraw-Hill.

Chey, W. D., & Wong, B. C. (2007). American College of Gastroenterology guideline on the management of *Helicobacter pylori* infection. *American Journal of Gastroenterology, 102*, 1808–1825.

Katz, P. O., Gerson, L. B., & Vela, M. F. (2013). Guidelines for the diagnosis and management of gastroesophageal reflux disease. *American Journal of Gastroenterology, 108,* 308–328.

North of England Dyspepsia Guideline Development Group. (2004, August 1). *Dyspepsia: Managing dyspepsia in adults in primary care.* Newcastle Upon Tyne, UK: University of Newcastle Upon Tyne.

Ranjan, P. (2012). Non-ulcer dyspepsia. *Journal of the Association of Physicians of India, 60* (Suppl.), 13–15.

HEAVY MENSTRUAL FLOW

Case Presentation: A 16-year-old female described a prolonged heavy menstrual flow with increased cramping over the past 8 days. This was unlike her normal menses, which were normal in the past.

INTRODUCTION TO COMPLAINT

Heavy menstrual bleeding can be caused by:

- Hormonal imbalance
- Uterine fibroid tumors
- Cervical polyps
- Endometrial polyps
- Infection
- Cervical cancer
- Endometrial cancer
- Intrauterine devices (IUDs)

HISTORY OF COMPLAINT

Symptomatology

Ask about the following characteristics of each symptom using open-ended questions:

- Onset (sudden or gradual)
- Chronology: when did this start to occur?
- Current situation (improving or deteriorating)
- Quality: describe the amount
- Timing (frequency, duration)
- Severity
- Precipitating and aggravating factors
- Relieving factors
- Associated symptoms
- Effects on daily activities
- Previous diagnosis of similar episodes
- Previous treatments
- Efficacy of previous treatments

Directed Questions to Ask

- How long have you had menstrual irregularities?
- Age of menarche (when you had your first menstrual period)?
- Duration of the menstrual period?

- Is the menstrual interval regular?
- What is the interval of your menstrual cycle?
- How old are you now?
- How saturated are the pads you use? Do you get clots, if yes, how big would the clots be?
- Dysmenorrhea?
- Intermenstrual bleeding, that is, spotting between your menstrual periods?
- Bleeding after intercourse?
- Have you experienced painful intercourse?
- Do you have excessive vaginal discharge? If so, describe the discharge.

Assessment: Cardinal Signs and Symptoms

- Dysmenorrhea
- Polymenorrhea
- Oligamenorrhea
- Menorrhagia
- Metorrhagia
- Postcoital bleeding
- Premenstrual syndrome

Medical History: General

- Allergies to medications
- Smoking or drinking alcohol
- Previous medical history or surgeries
- Medications
- Sexually active
- Last sexual encounter
- Birth control or barrier devices
- Last gynecological exam
- Family members with problems of heavy bleeding

Medical History: Specific to Complaint

- Start of menses
- Regularity of periods
- Color of flow
- Length of flow
- Number of pads used per day
- Bleeding between cycles
- Cramping, then and now
- Pregnancies
- Miscarriages or abortions
- Consistency of the bleeding now

PHYSICAL EXAMINATION

Vital Signs

- Temperature
- Pulse

- Respiration
- Blood pressure (BP)
- SpO$_2$ (oxygen saturation)

General Appearance

- Apparent state of health: The patient is quite pale. She is having cramping and heavy bleeding at the time of examination.
- Appearance of comfort or distress: The patient is in apparent distress on examination due to cramping of the abdomen and low back pain.
- Color: She is extremely pale.
- Nutritional status: She is 15 pounds overweight, 162 lbs; body mass index (BMI) 26.1.
- State of hydration: She is well hydrated as evidenced by good skin turgor.
- Hygiene: She is well dressed and kempt.
- Match between age and appearance: The patient appears her stated age of 16 years.
- Difficulty with gait or balance: There is no difficulty with gait or balance.

CASE STUDY

History

Questions	Response
Do you have allergies to medications?	*No*
Do you smoke cigarettes or drink alcohol?	*No*
Do you have a previous medical history or surgeries?	*No, no*
Do you use any medications?	*No*
How long have you had menstrual irregularities?	*Since my first period*
Age of menarche (when first got menstrual period)?	*11*
Duration of the menstrual period?	*5 to 7 days*
Is the menstrual interval regular?	*Yes*
What is the interval of your menstrual cycle?	*26 days*
How old are you now?	*16*
With heavy menstrual bleeding, how many pads or tampons do you use per day?	*I change my tampons every hour and always wear a pad for extra protection*
With the heavy bleeding do you experience large clots?	*Yes, there have been large clots for the past year, the size of a half dollar*
Dysmenorrhea?	*Yes, bad cramps*
Intermenstrual bleeding (i.e., spotting between your menstrual periods?	*No*

Questions	*Response*
When was your last gynecological exam?	*When I was 15 and the exam was normal*
Do any family members have problems with heavy bleeding?	*When my mom was my age she had heavy menstrual flow*
Are you sexually active?	*No (APN had doubts about this response)*
When was your last sexual encounter?	*A month ago. I had a boyfriend but we broke up.*
Do you use any type of birth control or barrier devices?	*No*
Bleeding after intercourse?	*No*
Do you experience painful intercourse? If so, is the discomfort within the vagina or deep within the abdomen?	*Deep*
Have you experienced vaginal discharge between periods?	*No discharge*
Was the onset of the bleeding gradual or sudden?	*Sudden*
What is the consistency of the bleeding now?	*Very heavy, with big clots of dark blood*
Have you had any fever?	*No*
Have you had any cramping?	*Yes*
Do you normally have cramps with your period?	*No*
On a scale of 0 to 10, rate your pain.	*3 or 4*
Have you ever been pregnant?	*No*
Do you have fatigue?	*Yes, very tired, sleeping a lot, don't feel like doing anything*
Have you had any nausea or vomiting?	*I feel queasy*
Any breast tenderness?	*No*
Is your abdomen tender?	*Yes, very*
Are you bleeding at this time?	*Yes*
How many days have you had the heavy bleeding?	*8 days*

Physical Examination Findings

- VITAL SIGNS: temperature 98.2°F, pulse 92, BP 110/70, respirations 20, SpO_2 98%
- GENERAL APPEARANCE: patient is a 16-year-old, well-developed, overweight, Caucasian female; skin is cold and clammy to touch; her height is 5′6″ and weight is 162 lbs; her BMI is 26.1.
- HEENT: head and neck are within normal limits; pupils equal, round, and reactive to light and accommodation (PERRLA); extraocular movements are intact. nonicteric sclerae. nares are patent; no edema or exudate of the turbinates are noted; all teeth present with no apparent gum hyperplasia; tonsils are normal; no redness or exudate are noted; neck range of motion is within normal limits. there is no lymph node enlargement on palpation; thyroid is not enlarged.
- CHEST: lungs are clear
- HEART: S1 and S2 are normal; no murmur, gallop, or rub noted
- ABDOMEN: excess fat in abdomen; tender to deep palpation, pain is worse in the right and left lower quadrants of abdomen; no distention is noted; suprapubic tenderness present upon examination
- BACK: pain and tenderness located in the lower back on palpation
- PELVIC: no discharge is noted; heavy bleeding and bloodclots noted; cervix is normal in color and round; extreme tenderness and pain are noted on cervical motion; the cervical os is closed; the uterus is enlarged and tenderness is noted in the posterior aspect of the abdomen; fundal height is noted at 4 cm; the hymen is not intact; palpation of the ovaries does elicit some tenderness bilaterally; the ovaries are noted to be 2 to 4 cm in size
- EXTREMITIES: within normal limits; no edema is noted

Specific to OB/GYN

- GENERAL: The patient is a 16-year-old female who is complaining of abdominal cramping with heavy menstrual flow for the past 8 days. The patient has a history of heavy menstrual periods; however, this is different from her normal menstrual periods. She is quite pale and her skin is cold and clammy. She is 5′6″ in height and weighs approximately 162 lbs. Her BMI is 26.1. She states she doesn't exercise and is not active in sports. She is an overachiever scholastically as evidenced by taking prerequisite classes in high school for entry into law school. She is disciplined in this endeavor and involved in her journal club.
- BREASTS: The patient states she has no tenderness or soreness and none is elicited on exam.
- ABDOMEN: The patient has excess fat on her abdomen. She is very tender to deep palpation, stating the pain is worse in the right and left lower quadrants of her abdomen. She raises her legs due to the pain elicited on deep palpation. There is no evidence of bloating or distention. When questioned about nausea or vomiting, the patient states "I have some queasiness." There is suprapubic tenderness also.
- BACK: She states she has pain in her lower back. She states this is a constant ache. She states that she had really bad lower back pain when I palpated her abdomen. She states the pain in her lower back, on a scale of 0 to 10, is a 3 or 4. The pain is made worse on palpation of the lower back.
- PELVIC: On general inspection, there is no discharge from the vagina; however large blood clots and heavy bleeding are noted. A pediatric speculum was used and the hymen is noted to be not intact. The cervix is normal in color and round. There is extreme tenderness noted in the cervical area on movement, and the patient complains of pain. The cervical os is closed. No discharge is noted from the cervical os. Vaginal mucosa appears normal. On bimanual exam the uterus is noted to be enlarged and tender in the posterior aspect. Fundal height is noted at 4 cm. Palpation of the ovaries reveal no masses, however, there is slight tenderness bilaterally. The ovaries are 2 to 4 cm in size.

DIFFERENTIAL DIAGNOSIS

Differential Diagnoses	PID	Spontaneous Abortion (Miscarriage)	Threatened Abortion	Ectopic Pregnancy	Fibroids/ Polyps
Dysmenorrhea	Rare	(+)	(+)	Common	Common
Abdominal pain/ cramping	Common	(+)	(+)	Common	Not a common complaint, unlikely
Uterus enlarged on examination	Rare	(+)	(+)	(+ or −)	Common
Painful uterus on examination	Rare	(+)	(+)	(+ or −)	(+ or −)
Painful cervix on examination	(+)	Rare	(+)	(+)	(−)
Fever	(+)	Rare	Rare	(−)	(−)
Acute bleeding in a normally regular menstrual cycle	Rare	(+)	(+)	Rare	Common
Nausea/vomiting	(+)	Common	(+)	Rare	Rare
Dizziness/fainting	Rare	Rare	(+)	(+)	Rare

DIAGNOSTIC EXAMINATIONS

Examinations	Procedure Code	Cost	Results
Complete blood count (CBC)	85025	$75	CBC: Typically has several parameters • White blood count (WBC): When an infection is present, the WBCs elevate in number • WBC differential: ■ Neutrophils: The most abundant of the white blood cells; respond more rapidly to areas of tissue injury and infection ■ Eosinophils: allergic or parasitic illnesses ■ Basophils: Will increase during the healing process ■ Monocytes: Second defense mechanism against bacterial and inflammatory illnesses; slower to respond than neutrophils but are bigger and can ingest larger organisms ■ Lymphocytes: Increased after chronic bacterial and viral infections

(continued)

Examinations	Procedure Code	Cost	Results
			• Red blood cells (RBCs): Carry O$_2$ from the lungs to the body • Hematocrit: This is the amount of space the RBCs take up in the blood • Hemoglobin: Carries oxygen and gives the RBCs their color; determines the ability of blood to carry oxygen throughout the body • Mean corpuscular volume: Shows the size of RBCs • MCH: Shows the amount of hemoglobin contained in the average RBC • MCHC: Measures the concentration of the hemoglobin in an average RBC • Platelets: The platelets play an important role in blood clotting. When bleeding occurs, the platelets swell, clump together, and form a stick plug that helps stop bleeding. If there are too few platelets, uncontrolled bleeding can occur. If there are too many, a blood clot can form in the artery.
Qualitative urine human chorionic gonadotropin (hCG) test	81025	$64	A urine pregnancy test is one of the easiest and less expensive laboratory and diagnostic studies to confirm or exclude a pregnancy. If a more sensitive test is needed, the serum hCG can be used.
Pelvic examination	89.26	$155	A pelvic examination can assist with determining a diagnosis by assessing and palpating the uterus, uterus size, cervix and cervical size, whether or not the cervical os is open or closed
Ultrasound transvaginal Ultrasound pelvic	76830 76856	$130	Can detect complications of pregnancy, such as ectopic pregnancy or a threatened abortion or absence of conception; cysts or polyps can be identified as well

CLINICAL DECISION MAKING

Case Study Analysis

The assessment on the patient is completed and data analysis is as follows: A 16-year-old female with an 8-day history of prolonged heavy menstrual flow and increased cramping that presents with a hematocrit level of 20. The patient had extreme tenderness on pelvic examination to include an enlarged uterus with the posterior part of uterus positive for tenderness. When the cervix was palpated, the patient was noted to have discomfort. Fundal height of the uterus is measured at 4 cm. A urine pregnancy test done on the patient is positive. The diagnosis is threatened abortion. A referral to OB/GYN is made as well as counseling the patient on birth control methods for the future.

Diagnosis: *Threatened abortion*

FURTHER READING

AAPC. (2013). *CPT code for pelvic exam.* Retrieved from http://www.aapc.com/memberarea/forums/showthread.php?t=44779

ARUP Laboratories. (2013). *Beta-hCG, urine qualitative.* Retrieved from http://www.aruplab.com/guides/ug/tests/0020229.jsp

Bickley, L. S., & Szilagyi, P. G. (2009). *Bates' guide to physical examination and history taking.* Philadelphia, PA: Lippincott Williams & Wilkins.

Dains, J. E., Bauman, L. C., & Scheibel, P. (2007). *Advanced health assessment and clinical diagnosis in primary care.* St. Louis, MO: Elsevier Mosby.

Healthcare Blue Book. (2013). *Healthcare blue book: Your free guide to fair healthcare pricing.* Retrieved from http://www.healthcarebluebook.com/page_Results.aspx?CatID=201

WebMD. (2012, August 6). *Complete blood count (CBC).* Retrieved from http://www.webmd.com/a-to-z-guides/complete-blood-count-cbc

HIP PAIN

Case Presentation: *A 66-year-old African American woman reports a complaint of hip pain from a fall she had 3 weeks ago.*

INTRODUCTION TO COMPLAINT

Hip pain can occur from a fall and subsequent damage to the hip joint. Damage can also occur from a number of causes includes sports-related injury, exercises, old age, overuse, and falls. Also, certain diseases lead to hip pain, including osteoarthritis, rheumatoid arthritis, avascular arthritis, and bone cancer.

Injuries That Cause Hip Pain

Hip Dislocation
- An injury to a joint in which the ends of the bones are forced from their normal positions
- This injury immobilizes the hip joint and results in sudden and severe pain

Hip Fracture
- Usually occurs in the joint area where the head of the femur is fractured. This results in extreme pain and immobility.
- Multiple medications

Hip Labral Tear
- Tear involves the labrum that follows the outside rim of the socket of the hip joint
- The labrum acts like a socket to hold the ball at the top of the femur in place

Compartment Syndrome
- Results from bleeding or swelling after an injury into a compartment space
- High pressure in compartment syndrome impedes the flow of blood to and from the affected tissues

Osteoporosis
- Causes bones to become weak and brittle so that a fall or even mild stresses like bending over or coughing can cause a fracture
- Physical findings include palpable tenderness over the area of compression fracture
- Osteoporosis-related fractures most commonly occur in the hip, wrist, or spine, especially in older people

Bursitis
- Affects the bursae
- Occurs when bursae become inflamed and patient experiences pain

Tendinitis
- Inflammation or irritation of a tendon
- Causes focal pain and tenderness just outside a joint due to trauma-related activities
- One of the most common sites is hip

Diseases That Cause Hip Pain

Osteoarthritis
- Most common form of arthritis
- Often called wear-and-tear arthritis
- Occurs when the protective cartilage on the ends of the bones wears down over time

Rheumatoid Arthritis
- Affects the synovial membranes, causing edema
- Results in bone erosion and damage to ligaments and tendons
- An autoimmune disorder

Paget's Disease
- Disrupts body's normal bone recycling process
- Old bone tissue is gradually replaced with new bone tissue
- Over time, the affected bones become fragile and can cause pain and tenderness

HISTORY OF COMPLAINT

Symptomatology

Ask about the following characteristics of each symptom using open-ended questions:

- Quality and severity of the pain
- Location
- Range of motion
- Relieving factors
- Radiation
- Ability to walk
- Gait and balance affected
- Able to complete activities of daily living
- Is the pain continuous or intermittent?
- What makes the pain worse: walking, bending, or extending the knee?
- Relief from pain with rest
- Medications or treatments tried
- Burning, cramping, or aching pain

Directed Questions to Ask

In addition to the general characteristics outlined above, additional characteristics of specific symptoms were elicited as follows:

- How is your balance?
- Are you able to walk straight?
- Are you able to bear weight on your both legs? Which legs hurt more when you walk?
- Are you able to raise your left hip?
- What about your right hip?
- Did you notice the shortening of any one leg?
- Did you notice any external rotation of your leg/hip?

- Do you have any redness or swelling?
- Did you notice any bulge in your inguinal area?
- Did you notice any lymph nodes in your groin area?
- Do you feel any pain in your groin area?
- Did you have any pain in your ischiogluteal area? Sciatica?
- Are you able to flex your hip? (bend your knee)
- Are you able to extend your hip? (lie face down, then bend your knee and lift it up)
- Are you able to abduct your leg? (lying flat, moving your leg away from the midline)
- Are you able to adduct your legs? (lying flat, bend your knee and move your lower leg toward the midline)
- Are you able to rotate the leg internally? (lying flat, bend your knee and turn your lower leg and foot away from the midline)

Assessment: Cardinal Signs and Symptoms

- Extreme localized pain in the affected area
- Inability to abduct or adduct affected limb
- Paresthesia
- Swelling or edema

Other Associated Symptoms

- Chills or fever
- Malaise
- Nausea or vomiting
- Pain or swelling or any joint pain
- Restricted or limited movement of any other joints

Medical History: General

- Obese with a 5-year history of hypertension controlled with medication
- Denies other significant history
- Has never fallen before
- Good general health

Medical History: Specific to Complaint

- Area is swollen and painful to touch
- Aching with occasional numbness and tingling
- Some relief with Motrin

PHYSICAL EXAMINATION

Vital Signs

- BP
- Pulse
- Respirations
- Temperature

General Appearance

- Body mass index (BMI)
- Height, weight
- Abdominal girth

Musculoskeletal

- Hip adduction decreased with less than 20%
- Hip abduction could not be determined due to pain
- Range of motion undetermined due to pain
- Patient refuses further examination due to pain

CASE STUDY

History

Question	Response
How is your general state of health?	*I am obese. I don't brush my teeth enough and have several cavities. My skin is warm and dry.*
Do you have any history of medical conditions like diabetes, high blood pressure, high cholesterol, or cancer?	*Yes, I have high blood pressure*
Did you have any heart problems or a history of cardiovascular disease?	*No*
Did you have any breathing or respiratory problems?	*No*
Did you have any stomach or gastric problems in the past?	*Yes, I have GERD*
Did you have any surgeries in the past? Any hospitalization?	*No*
Are you allergic to any medication, food, or plants? Any seasonal allergies?	*No*
Do you have any history of lupus, psoriasis, Lyme disease, gonococcal infection, rubella, or rheumatic fever?	*No*
Are your immunizations up to date?	*I don't know*
Do you currently use any medications that include any prescription medications?	*Yes, I take Prilosec for GERD and a calcium channel blocker and hydrochlorothiazide for hypertension*
Do you use any over-the-counter medications?	*No*
Did you use any herbal preparations or traditional therapies?	*I use Bio-freeze for my hip pain*
Do you have any weakness in any of your extremities?	*No*
Any changes in your activities?	*I am not able to wear my high-heel shoes now. I feel wobbly.*

Question	Response
Do you have any trauma, injury, or fracture of your hip before?	*No*
Do you have arthritis?	*I believe I have arthritis in my right knee. But no doctors told me that.*
Do you have any unsteady gait? Do you use any assistive devices?	*No*
Do you drink or smoke?	*No*
Do you have trouble falling asleep at night?	*No*
Are you sleeping more than usual, such as taking naps throughout the day?	*No*
Do you feel like your appetite has increased or decreased?	*No, I am obese*
Where do you live, and who lives with you? (Spouse, son, daughter).	*With my daughter and grandkids*
How well do get along with your household members?	*Good*

Physical Examination Findings

- VITAL SIGNS: temperature 98.6°F (oral); pulse 72 beats/min; respiration 24 beats/min; blood pressure 142/92 mmHg (supine), 138/90 mmHg (sitting), 138/92 mmHg (standing)
- GENERAL APPEARANCE: Older adult, obese, African American female, who was admitted due to syncope with a complaint of hip pain from a fall. She is in a fair state of health and concerned about the episode of her fainting spell. She is 5 feet 4 inches tall and weighs 213 pounds. Appears neat and clean, however, with poor dentition. Her appearance matches with her age. Her mood looks worried and anxious. Skin looks normal. Nutritional status is fair, drinks eight glasses of water per day. She has difficulty with gait or balance. States feeling wobbly when walking due to her obesity and right knee pain.
- ACCU-CHECK: random blood glucose 82
- SKIN: skin is warm and dry with no open lesions; quarter size, yellowish green old bruise on right hip
- CARDIAC EXAMINATION: EKG reveals normal sinus rhythm; echocardiogram was normal
- PULMONARY EXAMINATION: oxygen saturation, 96%; respirations regular and even. Lungs clear
- GASTRIC EXAMINATION: abdomen obese, soft, nontender; bowel sounds normoactive
- HIP/MUSCULOSKELETAL EXAMINATION:
  - Bilateral hips no swelling or deformity
  - Right hip has quarter size, yellowish green old bruise
  - Mild irritation and tenderness on internal rotation of the right hip
  - Hands with degenerative changes and stiffness
  - Right knee with moderate effusion and tenderness
  - Both feet have bunions
  - All other joints with good range of motion, no other deformity or swelling

DIFFERENTIAL DIAGNOSIS

Differential Diagnosis	Muscle Injury/Strain	Compartment syndrome	Hip Fracture	Labral Tear	Tendon Injury
Location of the pain	Hip muscle pain	Persistent deep ache in the hip and right knee	Pain in the hip, lower groin	Groin pain, buttocks and thigh pain	Pain in the affected area where the injured tendon is located or may radiate out from the joint area
Quality of the pain	Muscle tightness, weakness	Pain that seems greater than expected for the severity of the injury, bruising	Severe pain and swelling	Sharp deep pain	Tenderness, redness, warmth/ swelling near the injured tendon
Course of the pain	Inability to fully stretch the injured muscle	Persistent everyday pain, hurts when pressure is applied to the area	Inability to walk or move hips, abnormal appearance and shortening of the broken leg	Worse with extension, episodes of deep clicking, feeling of hip giving away	Pain and stiffness may be worse during night or when getting up in the morning; pain may increase with activity
Involvement of trauma	+	+	+	+ or −	+

DIAGNOSTIC EXAMINATION

Examination	Procedure Code	Cost	Results
Plain x-ray	M25.559	$350	An x-ray can reveal deterioration of the structure of the hip, an excess of bone on the femoral head or neck and the acetabular rim. X-ray anterior–posterior and lateral view showed no abnormalities
CT scan	M12.559	$1500	CT scan provides digital images of the body using a thin x-ray beam to produce a more detailed, cross-sectional image of the body
Compartment pressure measurement	20950	$150	Insert a needle into the area of suspected compartment syndrome while an attached pressure monitor records the pressure. A plastic catheter can also be inserted to monitor the compartment pressure continuously. Compartment measurement within 20 mmHg of diastolic pressure is an indication of fasciotomy.

CLINICAL DECISION MAKING
Case Study Analysis

The provider performs the assessment and physical examination on a 66-year-old female and reports the following data: the diagnosis of hip pain evidenced by bruise due to fall; physical examination revealed limited internal rotation of the right hip, with tenderness. For the confirmation of diagnoses, laboratory diagnostic tests of complete blood count and blood chemistry, compartment pressure measurement, and pelvic x-ray must be done.

> ***Diagnosis:*** *Hip pain due to trauma and fall*

FURTHER READING

Bickley, L. (2013). *Bate's guide to physical examination and history taking* (11th ed.). Philadelphia, PA: Lippincott Williams and Wilkins.

Dains, J. E., Baumann, L. C., & Scheibel, P. (2007). *Advanced health assessment and clinical diagnosis in primary care* (3rd ed.). St. Louis, MO: Mosby Elsevier.

OrthoInfo, American Academy of Orthopedic Surgeons. (2009, October). *Compartment syndrome.* Retrieved from http://orthoinfo.aaos.org/topic.cfm?topic=a00204

WebMD. (2012, August 13). *Hip pain: causes and treatment.* Retrieved from http://www.webmd.com/pain-management/guide/hip-pain-causes-and-treatment

KNEE PAIN

Case Presentation: A 56-year-old teacher presents to your clinic with a complaint of right knee pain for 2 weeks after playing soccer.

INTRODUCTION TO COMPLAINT

Knee pain is a common complaint in primary care. Most common cause is osteoarthritis (OA).

Acute Knee Pain

- The knee is a joint that is frequently injured in weight-bearing sports
  - Medial/lateral meniscus injury
    - Medial more common than lateral
  - Medial/lateral collateral ligament injury (MCL/LCL)
    - Medial more common than lateral
  - Anterior/posterior cruciate ligament injury (ACL/PCL)
    - Anterior more common than posterior
- Gout
- Fracture

Chronic Knee Pain

- Common site of OA in population older than 50 years

Uncommon But Not to Be Missed Etiology

- Septic arthritis
- Rheumatoid arthritis (RA)
- Malignancy

Consider Mixed Etiology

- Acute injury with OA
- Systemic condition with OA or acute injury

Consider Age of Patients

- Pediatric population
  - Osgood–Schlatters disease
  - Patellar tendinitis (jumper's knee)
  - Osteochondritis dissecans
  - Patellar subluxation
- Young adult
  - Patellofemoral syndrome (PFS)
    - Collection of symptoms
    - More common in women than in men

- Can be due to overuse (repetitive microtrauma)
- Can be due to misalignment: Q angle, quadriceps weakness, patella cartilage damage
- Chondromalacia patellae
  - Soft cartilage behind the knee
  - Requires biopsy of cartilage for definitive diagnosis
- Patellar tendinitis (jumper's knee)
- Reiter's syndrome
- RA
  - Morning stiffness longer than 30 minutes
- Bursitis (pes anserine)
- Septic knee
- Systemic disease (i.e., lupus)
- Older adult
  - OA
    - Morning stiffness improves with activity
  - Gout/pseudogout
  - Baker's cyst
  - Septic knee
  - Systemic disease

Consider Location of Pain

Have patient point to where pain is with one finger.

- Anterior knee pain
  - Osgood–Schlatters disease
  - Patellar tendinitis (jumper's knee)
  - Patellar subluxation
  - Prepatellar bursitis
  - PFS
  - Chondromalacia patellae
  - OA
- Posterior knee pain
  - PCL tear
  - Baker's cyst
- Medial knee pain
  - MCL injury
  - Medial meniscus injury
  - Bursitis (pes anserine)
- Lateral knee pain
  - LCL injury
  - Lateral meniscus injury
  - Iliotibial band syndrome

Consider Referred Pain

- Hip
- Ankle
- Neuropathy
- Malignance

HISTORY OF COMPLAINT

Symptomatology

Ask about the following characteristics of each symptom using open-ended questions:

Start with history and medication use

- Previous knee pain/injury
- Systemic disease (rheumatoid conditions, diabetes mellitus [DM])
- Knee surgical history
- Allergies (medication and seasonal)
- Medications currently used daily and as needed
  - Prescription
  - Over the counter, including herbal and traditional therapies
  - What is the effect of the medication used on the current pain?

The following characteristics of symptoms should be elicited and explored:

- Acute onset with injury
  - What did the pain feel like at onset?
    - Pop/snap consider ACL injury
  - Was there immediate swelling and difficulty with ambulation?
    - ACL tear
    - Dislocation of patella
    - Fracture
  - Able to keep doing activity or did you have to stop due to pain?
  - What was the mechanism of injury?
    - Type of activity you were doing and on what surface?
    - Was there direct contact?
    - Direction of force: hyperextension; valgus stress (blow to lateral knee)—MCL; varus stress (blow to medial knee)—LCL; blow to anterior knee—PCL, patella subluxation/dislocation
    - Twisting injury: ACL, meniscus injury, patellar subluxation/dislocation
    - Sudden stop: ACL
- Gradual onset without known injury
  - OA
  - Systemic etiology
  - Malignancy
- Current associated symptoms
  - Locking, clicking, catching
    - Meniscus injury
    - Loose bodies within joint space
  - Knee giving way
    - Meniscus injury
    - ACL tear
    - Loose bodies within joint space
    - Patellar subluxation
  - Knee locks
    - Meniscus injury
  - Radiating pain
- Location of pain (see Consider Location of Pain on previous page)
- Current situation (improving or deteriorating)

Directed Questions to Ask

- Was the onset of pain sudden or gradual?
- If chronic knee pain—is this pain worse than your usual pain?
- What brought you in today?
- What were you doing when the pain started?
- Was there an injury? If so, what was the mechanism of injury?

- Were you able to keep playing after injury?
- What is your level of pain on a 0 to 10 scale now?
  - What makes the pain worse?
  - Does the pain keep you awake at night/awaken you from sleep?
- Where is the pain? With one finger point to where the pain is.
- Describe the pain.
  - Popping, clicking, catching, buckling
- Do you have pain with range of motion (ROM)?
  - Is ROM limited?
- Is there associated weakness?
- Does pain radiate?
- Do you have numbness, tingling in feet?
- Have you had a previous diagnosis of knee pain?
  - When
  - Frequency (are episodes increasing?)
- Previous treatments
  - Efficacy of previous treatments
- Was imaging done?
  - Findings

Assessment: Cardinal Signs and Symptoms of Adjacent Systems

Hip
- Hip pain
- Hip injury
- Decreased ROM of hip
- Past history of hip problems

Ankle
- Ankle pain
- Recent ankle injury
- Decreased ROM ankle

Calf
- Calf pain
- Recent calf injury
- Calf lesions/discoloration

Associated symptoms
- Fever
- Systemic symptoms
- Paresthesias distal foot

PHYSICAL EXAMINATION
Vital Signs

- Temperature
- Pulse
- Respiration
- Blood pressure (BP)

General Appearance

- Apparent state of health
- Appearance of comfort or distress
- Color and temperature of skin

- Nutritional status
- State of hydration
- Hygiene
- Match between appearance and stated age
- Difficulty with gait or balance

Knee
- Inspect (compare to unaffected knee)
  - Position in which patient is holding knee
  - Presence of effusion
  - Presence of erythema or lesions
- Palpate
  - Presence of warmth
  - Bony tenderness: knee
    - Patella
    - Tibial plateau
  - Tenderness along MCL, LCL, popliteal, medial, or lateral joint lines
  - Tenderness or atrophy of distal quadriceps
- Evaluate ROM of knee
  Observe for evidence of pain with ROM and if symmetrical right to left
  - Flexion 140 plus or minus
  - Extension 0 (not uncommon to hyperextend to minus 5 to 6)
- Perform tests
  - Ballottement and/or bulge sign to determine whether effusion is present
  - McMurray test to detect meniscus injury
  - Lachman test to determine integrity of ACL (most sensitive test for ACL injury)
  - Drawer test to determine whether there is instability of ACL or PCL
  - Varus stress test to determine stability of LCL
    - Push calf laterally (abduction)
  - Valgus stress test to determine stability of MCL
    - Push calf medially (adduction)
- Evaluate ROM of hips: Does patient have pain with ROM of hips?
- Evaluate distal neurological status if complaints of paresthesias

CASE STUDY

History

- History: positive for controlled hypertension (HTN); OA diagnosed 3 years prior; negative for systemic illness, cardiac disease, DM
- Negative surgical history
- Medications: Lisinopril 10 mg daily; currently using over-the-counter ibuprofen 400 mg two to three times per day without relief
- No known drug allergies

Question	Response
Was the onset sudden or gradual?	*Sudden onset*
If chronic knee pain—is this pain worse than your usual pain?	*Yes, since soccer injury*
What brought you in today?	*Pain is not improving after 2 weeks*
What were you doing when it started?	*Playing soccer*

Question	*Response*
What was the mechanism of injury?	*Another player ran into lateral right knee*
Were you able to keep playing after injury?	*Yes, but it hurt a bit*
What is your level of pain on a 0 to 10 scale?	*Initially 3 to 4 on 10, today 5 to 6 on 10*
What makes pain worse?	*Walking*
Describe pain	*Medial knee pain with most activities*
Popping, clicking, catching, buckling in the knee	*Yes, occasionally will give way (baseline)*
Does the pain keep you awake at night/ awaken you from sleep?	*Not really*
Do you have pain with ROM?	*Especially with flexion*
Is ROM limited?	*Yes*
Is there associated weakness?	*Not that I know of*
Do you have numbness, tingling in your feet?	*No, that seems okay*
Does pain radiate?	*Sometimes to back of knee with walking*
Do you have fever or sign of infection?	*I feel OK other than my knee*
Have you had a previous diagnosis of knee pain?	*Yes, I was told I had arthritis.*
When?	*Three years ago when first started hurting and "giving way"*
Are episodes increasing?	*Do not have episodes, have mild pain most of the time*
Have you had previous treatments?	*Tylenol and nonsteroidal anti-inflammatory drugs (NSAIDs) usually help but not now*
Was imaging done?	*They did an x-ray and told me that I had arthritis in my knee*

Physical Examination Findings

- VITAL SIGNS: temperature 98.6°F; respiratory rate (RR) 16, heart rate (HR) 82 (regular), blood pressure (BP) 138/784
- GENERAL APPEARANCE: well developed, appropriate for age; gait favors right leg
- KNEE
  - No effusion, erythema, or lesions
  - Tender to palpation along MCL. No tenderness at patellar tendon, popliteal, LCL, or joint lines
  - No bony tenderness of patella or tibial plateau
  - Decreased and painful flexion at 90%
  - Instability with valgus stress test
  - Negative McMurray, Lachman, and Drawer tests

- Hip examination unremarkable
  - Symmetrical bilaterally
  - Full ROM without pain
  - Negative Patrick test
- Calf and ankle examination unremarkable
  - No erythema, effusion, warmth, tenderness, lesions
  - Full ROM without pain
- Extremities sensation intact distal foot

DIFFERENTIAL DIAGNOSIS

Differential Diagnosis	MCL/LCL Sprain	ACL/PCL	Meniscus Injury	Fracture	OA	Gout	Bursitis	Septic Joint
History of trauma	Positive	Positive	Positive	Positive	Negative	Negative	Negative	Negative
Onset	Sudden	Sudden	Sudden or gradual	Sudden	Gradual	Gradual	Gradual	Gradual
Knee pain	Positive	Positive	Positive	Positive	Positive	Positive	Positive	Positive
Unable to bear weight	Negative	Positive or negative	Negative	Positive	Negative	Negative	Negative	Positive or negative
Decreased and painful ROM	Positive	Positive	Positive or negative	Positive	Positive or negative	Positive or negative	Positive or negative	Positive
Bony tenderness	Negative	Negative	Negative	Positive	Negative	Negative	Negative	Negative
Medial or lateral pain	Positive	Negative	Positive	Positive	Positive or negative	Positive or negative	Positive or negative	Positive
Anterior or posterior pain	Negative	Positive	Positive or negative	Positive	Positive or negative	Positive or negative	Positive or negative	Positive
Locking, catching sensation	Negative	Negative	Positive	Negative	Positive or negative	Negative	Negative	Positive or negative
Knee giving way	Negative	Positive	Positive or negative	Positive or negative	Positive or negative	Negative	Negative	Positive or negative
Effusion	Positive or negative	Positive or negative	Negative	Positive	Negative	Positive or negative	Positive or negative	Positive
Erythema and warmth	Negative	Negative	Negative	Negative	Negative	Positive or negative	Positive or negative	Positive
Fever	Negative	Negative	Negative	Negative	Negative	Negative	Negative	Positive

DIAGNOSTIC EXAMINATION

- No laboratory examinations were indicated because there was no evidence of infection.
- Imaging was indicated per Pittsburgh and Ottawa Rules due to history of:
  - Age older than 55
  - Direct trauma
  - Inability to flex to 90%
- Radiograph showed osteophytes indicative of OA with possible loose body at medial aspect otherwise negative.

CLINICAL DECISION MAKING

Case Study Analysis

The APN performs history and physical examination on the patient and finds the following pertinent positives and negatives to rule out the differential.

The pertinent positive history findings are:

- History of age older than 55
- History of previous diagnosis of OA of the right knee with positive radiograph x-ray findings
- History of knee occasionally "giving way"
- History of recent direct blow to lateral right knee
- History of pain at time but able to keep playing soccer
- Describes pain along MCL with occasional clicking and locking

The pertinent negative history findings are:

- Was able to keep playing after injury (although it was painful)
- Denies fever or systemic symptoms
- Denies anterior, posterior knee pain
- Denies clicking, popping
- Denies hip pain
- Denies radiating pain or paresthesias

The pertinent positive physical examination findings are:

- Compensated gait favoring right knee
- Mild tenderness to palpation along MCL
- Decreased and painful flexion of right knee
- Instability with valgus stress test

The pertinent negative physical examination findings are:

- Normal vital signs, no fever
- No bony tenderness of patella or tibial plateau
- No tenderness along patellar tendon, popliteal, LCL, or joint lines
- No warmth, erythema
- Negative ballottement; bulge; and negative Lachman, Drawer, and McMurray tests
- No instability with Varus stress test

Diagnosis: Right knee MCL sprain in the setting of OA

FURTHER READING

Dains, J. E., Baumann, L. C., & Scheibel, P. (2012). Chapter 20. *Advanced health assessment and clinical diagnosis in primary care* (4th ed.). Elsevier.

EMRA: The Emergency Medicine Residents' Association. (2009). *Pittsburgh decision rules and Ottawa knee rules.* Retrieved from http://www.emra.org/content.aspx?id=861

Family Practice Notebook. (2011). *Acute knee pain.* Retrieved from http://www.fpnotebook.com /Ortho/Sx/ActKnPn.htm

Meredith, P. V., & Moran, N. M. (2000). *Adult primary care.* Philadelphia, PA: W.B. Saunders Company.

Seidel, H. M., Ball, J. W., Dains, J. E., Flynn, J. A., Solomon, B. S., & Stewart, R. W. (2011). *Mosby's guide to physical examination* (7th ed., pp. 681–683). St. Louis, MO: Mosby Elsevier.

LOW BACK PAIN

Case Presentation: *A 35-year-old male painter presents to your clinic with the complaint of low back pain. He recalls lifting a 5-gallon paint can and felt an immediate pull in the lower right side of his back. This happened 2 days ago and he had the weekend to rest, but after taking Motrin and using heat, he has not seen any improvement. He is having some right leg pain but no bowel or bladder changes. His pain is sharp, stabbing, and he scored it as a 9 on a scale of 0 to 10. He had a similar incident approximately 5 years ago but made a complete recovery.*

INTRODUCTION TO COMPLAINT

Acute low back pain is a common problem seen in primary care practices. Most low back pain can affects approximately 80% of the population between the ages of 25 and 45 years. Fortunately, 90% of back injuries are benign and account for the fifth most common visit in primary care. Some of the important characteristics of low back pain that are critical to making the correct diagnosis are:

- Localized pain that is worse with moving due to muscle pain
- Trauma may cause a fracture and requires an x-ray
- Radiating pain into the leg along a dermatone indicates a ruptured disc
- Loss of bowel or bladder function indications an emergency
- Back pain that is continuous and associated with a history of cancer requires diagnostic testing to rule out malignancy

HISTORY OF COMPLAINT

Symptomatology

Ask about the following characteristics of each symptom using open-ended questions:

- Chronology/onset/mechanism of injury
- Current situation (improving or deteriorating)
- Location
- Radiation
- Quality
- Timing (frequency, duration)
- Severity
- Precipitating and aggravating factors
- Relieving factors
- Associated factors
- Effects on daily living

- Previous low back injury or pain
- Previous treatments
- Efficacy of treatments
- Social history and lifestyle habits

Directed Questions to Ask

- What was the onset of your symptoms?
- What was the mechanism of injury? (without trauma may suggest serious disease)
- How did this occur?
- Where is your pain specifically? Point with one finger.
- Specifically ask about duration of pain; pain is considered chronic if it persists for more than 6 to 9 weeks.
- Are you having any numbness or tingling?
- Are you having any radiating pain?
- On a scale from 0 to 10 with 10 being the worst, could you rate your pain?
- Are you having any bowel or bladder issues? Difficulty with urination or going to the bathroom to have a bowel movement?
- Any difficulty with sleep?
- Any problems with sitting?
- Any problems with walking?
- Have you ever suffered a similar back problem like this before today? If so, when? What kind of treatments have you had in the past?
- Are you taking any medication for this problem? If so, what?
- Have tried any other home self-care remedies? If so, what?
- Are you allergic to any medications?

Assessment: Cardinal Signs and Symptoms

Any history of radiculopathy, foot drop, or bowel/bladder changes needs immediate attention and possibly an MRI and referral to a neurosurgeon.

Abdomen
- Pain
- Rectal bleeding
- Bowel linkage

Urinary
- Urinary linkage or incontinence
- Painful urination

Neurological
- Radiculopathy
- Foot drop
- Motor weakness of lower extremities

Other
- Fever
- Rash over one side of back (shingles)
- Malaise
- Enlarged lymph nodes in groin
- Pelvic pain or discharge (females)

Medical History: General

- Age
- Allergies
- Medications currently used (prescription, birth control pills [BCPs], and over-the-counter vitamins or medications)
- Herbal and home therapies
- Supplements
- Level of daily activity
- Physical exercise
- Lifestyle questions (smoking, alcohol, and recreational drugs)
- Other medical conditions
- Previous hospitalizations or surgeries

Medical History: Specific to Complaint

- Previous back injury, including motor vehicle accident (MVA) or work-related injury
- Previous back surgeries
- History of scoliosis or lordosis
- Increased pain with sitting, standing, or sleeping
- Occupation
- Hobbies or sport activities
- Second job

PHYSICAL EXAMINATION

Vital Signs

- Temperature; fever is an ominous sign
- Pulse
- Blood pressure
- SpO_2 (oxygen saturation)
- Respiration

General Appearance

- Apparent state of health
- Observe general gait for signs of limping
- Guarding or coordination problems while walking are important to note and suggest a possible neurological problem
- Appearance of comfort versus distress
- Overall muscle tone, alignment, and abnormalities

Lumbar Spine

Inspect
- Symmetrical checking for scoliosis, kyphosis, or lordosis
- Swelling
- Masses
- Discoloration
- Signs of infection
- Bruising of the skin

Palpate
- Tenderness, noting specific location and muscle spasms

Range of Motion
- Check forward flex
- Side to side bending
- Twisting and extension of the back
- Carefully watch the patient as they move on and off the examination table

Strength
Check lower extremity strength by asking the patient to push or lift knee up against the examiner's hand

- Watch for weakness or limitations with the range-of-motion (ROM) activities
- Have patient perform a push-up lying prone on the table and arch back leaving stomach on the table to see how flexible lower lumbar region is
- While patient is still on stomach, bring heel to buttocks
- On back, perform a knee-to-chest activity
- Watch the abdominal muscles when the patient sits up
- Check the gait by asking the patient to walk normally
- Walk on toes
- Walk on heel

Neurological
- Check lower extremity deep tendon reflexes (DTRs)
- Check sensory neurological tests by checking dermatomes

Special Test
- Straight leg raises (SLRs): Elevate each leg while the patient is lying down; if pain is indicated between 30 degrees and 60 degrees, this indicates a positive SLR and could be diagnostic of a herniated disc

Vascular
- Pedal pulses and leg swelling

Rectal Examination
- Indicated if patient presents with a history of falling on tailbone, rectal bleeding, or you suspect a malignancy.

Pelvic Examination
- Indicated if you suspect a gynecological problem, such as pelvic inflammatory disease

CASE STUDY
History

Question	Response
What was the onset of your symptoms?	*Abrupt*
What was the mechanism of injury?	*Lifting a heavy object (5 gallons of paint)*
How did this occur?	*Lifting a heavy object (5 gallons of paint)*
Where is your pain specifically?	*Right lower back*

Question	Response
Specifically how long have you had this pain?	*2 days*
Are you having any numbness or tingling?	*No*
Are you having any radiating pain?	*Yes, down the right leg*
On a scale from 0 to 10 with 10 being the worse, could you rate your pain?	*9*
Are you having difficulty with urination or any bowel changes?	*No*
Any difficulty with sleep?	*Some, when I turn over in bed*
Any problems with sitting?	*Not so much*
Any problems with walking?	*I am walking with a slight limp*
Have you ever suffered a similar back problem?	*Yes, about 5 years ago*
If so, when? What kind of treatments have you had in the past?	*It just resolved on its own*
What is your occupation? Full time or part time?	*Full-time painter*
Do you have any hobbies or sport activities?	*Coach my son's fifth-grade baseball team*
Do you have a second job?	*No*
Are you taking any medication for this problem?	*Motrin*
Have you tried any other home remedies? If so, what?	*Yes, I used a heating pad on it*
Are you allergic to any medications?	*No*

Physical Examination Findings

- VITAL SIGNS: 98.4°F, respiratory rate (RR) 16, heart rate (HR) 82, blood pressure (BP) 120/64, O_2 saturation 98%
- GENERAL APPEARANCE: well-developed healthy 35-year-old male; no gross deformities.
- CHEST: Lungs are clear in all fields. Heart S1, S2 no murmur, gallop, or rub.
- MUSCULATURE: No obvious deformities, masses, or discoloration. Palpable pain noted at the right lower lumbar region. No palpable spasms. ROM limited to forward bending 10 inches from floor; able to bend side to side but had difficulty twisting and going into extension. SLRs were negative
- NEUROLOGY: DTRs 2+ lower extremity (LE), SLR negative; sensory neurology intact to light touch and patient able to toe and heel walk. Gait was stable and no limping noted.

DIFFERENTIAL DIAGNOSIS

Differential Diagnosis	Lumbar Strain	Herniated Disc	Sacroiliac	Osteoarthritis	Malignancies
Onset	Abrupt	Either	Abrupt	Gradual	Gradual
Duration	< 2 weeks	Varies	Acute symptoms	Many years	Many years
Location	Lumbar region	Lumbar or thoracic region	Buttocks region	Lumbar region	Varies depending on location of malignancy
Pain	Can radiate	Can radiate	Can radiate	Can vary	Can vary
Numbness and tingling	Sometimes	Often	Sometimes	Not often	Varies
Bowel or bladder changes	No changes	Possible changes	No changes	No changes	Possible changes
DTR	Normal	Possible asymmetrical	Normal	Normal	Possible asymmetrical
Toe and heel walking	Normal	Difficulty depending on the location of the herniation	Difficulty	Normal	Normal
SLR	Normal	Abnormal or positive	Normal	Normal	Normal

DIAGNOSTIC EXAMINATION

Examination	Procedure Code	Cost	Results
Complete blood count (CBC), determination of erythrocyte sedimentation rate	85025	$15 to $25	Used to confirm the diagnosis of infection or malignancy
Plain-film radiographs, oblique views of the spine	72010	$150 to $175	Inexpensive and easily obtained. It provides two-dimensional view of motion and evidence of trauma
MRI	75571	$1600 to $1700	Superior contrast resolution with disadvantages being: it is a costly diagnostic test; it interacts with metals in the body

(*continued*)

Examination	Procedure Code	Cost	Results
CT scanning	72192	$300 to $700	Detects abnormal tissue; it is a useful technique for planning areas for radiotherapy and biopsies Can also provide valuable data on the patient's vascular condition, bone diseases, bone density, and the state of the patient's spine

CLINICAL DECISION MAKING
Case Study Analysis

A lumbar strain is based on history and clinical findings. A complete history may suggest the cause of the acute low back pain based on the mechanism of injury. If there is no obvious history of trauma or physical activities, it is important to consider other diagnostic tests to rule out pathology. No x-rays are indicated for minor low back pain, but if symptoms persist, x-rays, CT scan, and MRI are often considered.

Any systemic disease or neurological involvement might require further tests and possibly a referral to an appropriate specialist.

Diagnosis: Lumbar strain

FURTHER READING

Buckup, K. (2008). *Clinical tests for the musculoskeletal system.* Stuttgart, Germany: Georg Thieme Verlag.

Hattam, P., & Smeatham, A. (2010). *Special tests in musculoskeletal examination.* London, UK: Churchill Livingstone Elsevier.

Michigan Quality Improvement Consortium (MQIC). (2008). *Management of acute low back pain.* Southfield, MI: MQIC.

Rhoads, J., & Petersen, S. (2013). *Advanced health assessment and diagnostic reasoning* (2nd ed.). Sudbury, MA: Jones & Bartlett.

Seller, R., & Symons, A. (2012). *Differential diagnosis of common complaints* (6th ed.). Philadelphia, PA: Elsevier.

LOWER EXTREMITY EDEMA

Case Presentation: A healthy appearing 52-year-old gentleman presents with 2 weeks of increasing bilateral lower leg edema.

INTRODUCTION TO COMPLAINT

The most common causes of lower extremity edema are as follows:

- Venous stasis
- Congestive heart failure
- Renal failure
- Liver failure
- Obstruction of lymphatics due to ascites from tumor
- Fluid overload from excessive intravenous (IV) rehydration

HISTORY OF COMPLAINT

Symptomatology

Ask about the following characteristics of each symptom using open-ended questions:

- Onset (sudden or gradual)
- Chronology
- Current situation (improving or deteriorating)
- Location
- Severity
- Precipitating and aggravating factors
- Relieving factors
- Associated symptoms
- Effects on daily activities
- Previous diagnosis of similar episodes
- Previous treatments
- Efficacy of previous treatments

Directed Questions to Ask

- Was the onset sudden or gradual?
- Do you have any fevers?
- Do you have any pain?
- Is it hard to walk?
- Do you have any dyspnea?

- Do you have a cough?
- Have you started any new medications?
- What surgeries have you had?
- Do you have a history of any liver disease?
- Cardiac disease?
- Renal disease?
- Any history of malignancies?
- Any swollen lymph nodes?
- Previous lymph node dissection?
- Any recent prolonged travel?
- Recent insect bites/infections?
- Any history of intravenous drug abuse (IVDA), if so, how recent and where?
- Prolonged sitting?
- Recent cast/splints?
- Any recent surgeries?
- Any history of coagulopathies/family history?
- Previous pregnancy or premenstrual edema?
- Diet and/or history of malnutrition?
- Do you have a rash?

Assessment: Cardinal Signs and Symptoms

In addition to the general characteristics outlined above, additional characteristics of specific symptoms should be elicited, as follows:

Chest
- Jugular vein distension
- Lung sounds/evidence of pulmonary congestion
- Chest wall lesions spider angiomata
- Heart murmurs, diastolic gallop (S3)

Abdomen Examination
- Pain
- Shifting dullness or fluid wave
- Distension or ascites

Lower Extremity Examination
- Stasis dermatitis
- Pattern of edema pitting or nonpitting, bilateral, or unilateral
- Nausea or vomiting
- Pedal pulses
- Evidence of isolated warmth redness or pain

Other Associated Symptoms
- Fever
- Malaise
- Nausea or vomiting
- Periorbital edema
- Skin exam with spider angiomata

Medical History: General

- Medical conditions and surgeries
- Allergies (seasonal as well as others)

- Medication currently used (prescription and over-the-counter [OTC] medicine)
- Herbal preparations and traditional therapies

Medical History: Specific to Complaint

- Frequent episodes related to activity or nonactivity
- Congestive heart failure
- Renal disease
- Hypertension
- Trauma to the lower extremities
- History of vascular surgeries
- History of methicillin-resistant *Staphylococcus aureus* (MRSA)

PHYSICAL EXAMINATION

Vital Signs

- Temperature
- Pulse
- Respiration
- SpO$_2$ (oxygen saturation)
- Blood pressure (BP)

General Appearance

- Apparent state of health
- Appearance of comfort or distress with gait and respirations
- Color of skin
- Nutritional status
- State of hydration
- Hygiene
- Match between appearance and stated age

Lower Extremity Examination: Inspection

- Groin, assess for inguinal adenopathy
- Assess pulses and bruits of femoral artery
- Describe as firm or soft, fixed, or mobile
- Assess for femoral hernia
- Assess in males for scrotal edema
- Inspect thigh looking for warmth, tenderness, and asymmetrical girth
- Assess popliteal fossa for popliteal pulse pulsatile or enlarged/aneurysmal
- Color of lower extremity
- Assess color of legs in dependent or raised position
- Is there asymmetric leg swelling, and if so, to what level
- Dilated or varicose superficial veins
- Hair pattern or lack of
- Observe for ulceration of skin
- Assess for dorsalis pedis artery
- Assess for posterior tibial artery
- Nail growth

Lower Extremity Examination: Associated Systems for Assessment

- A complete assessment should include the respiratory system and abdomen

CASE STUDY

History

Question	Response
Was the onset sudden or gradual?	*It was gradual*
Do you have any pain?	*No, but my legs ache*
If 10 is the worst pain you have ever had, what number is this pain	*2/10*
Do you have any shortness of breath?	*A little, only with steep long stairs*
Do you have a cough?	*No*
Do you have any chest discomfort or pain?	*No*
Do you have a rash?	*No*
Do you have fatigue?	*Yes, but I always feel that way*
Do you have fevers?	*No*
Do you have a sense of one leg being more uncomfortable?	*No*
Do you have any nausea or vomiting?	*No*
Have you had any changes in your medication?	*Sort of*

Physical Examination Findings

- VITAL SIGNS: 98.9°F; RR 18; HR 88, regular; BP 156/102; pulse oximetry 97%
- GENERAL APPEARANCE: well-developed, heavy but healthy-appearing gentleman with normal voice in no acute distress
- CARDIOVASCULAR: no jugular vein (JV) distension, faint S3 appreciable. +3 femoral pulses equal, no bruits, dorsalis pedis pulse +2 equal right/left, posterior tibial pulse difficult to palpate due to edema
- CHEST: breath sounds equal, faint crackles in right and left bases, equal excursion, no fremitus, no egophony, no retractions, rate even and unlabored
- ABDOMEN: large, obese, no rashes or skin changes, no tenderness, rebound, or guarding; no appreciable fluid shift
- LOWER EXTREMITIES: no appreciable inguinal adenopathy, no hernia, no scrotal edema, skin without rashes, lesions, or excoriations; without unilateral pain, swelling, or warmth; has symmetrical edema up to about 6 cm below knee, increasing distally

DIFFERENTIAL DIAGNOSIS

Differential Diagnosis	Deep Vein Thrombosis	Venous Insufficiency	Cellulitis	Lymphedema	Heart Failure
Onset	Either	Gradual	Abrupt	Gradual	Gradual
Fever	No	No	Possible	No	No

Differential Diagnosis	Deep Vein Thrombosis	Venous Insufficiency	Cellulitis	Lymphedema	Heart Failure
Skin changes	Yes	Yes	Yes	No	No
Skin erythema/warmth	Yes	No	Yes	No	No
Edema	Unilateral	Bilateral	Unilateral	Either	Bilateral
Dyspnea	No	No	No	No	Possible
Chest discomfort	No	No	No	No	Possible
Jugular vein distension	No	No	No	No	Possible
Abdominal distension	No	No	No	No	Rare
Fatigue	No	Possible	No	No	Possible
Cough	No	No	No	No	Common
Lymphadenopathy	No	No	Possible	Yes	No

DIAGNOSTIC EXAMINATION

Examination	Procedure Code	Cost	Results
Transthoracic stress echo, complete with contrast EKG	93351	$1400 to $2500	• Evaluates all four chambers of the heart • Determines strength of the heart, the condition of the heart valves, the lining of the heart (the endocardium), and the aorta • Detects a heart attack, enlargement, or hypertrophy of the heart, infiltration of the heart with an abnormal substance • Detects weakness of the heart; cardiac tumors; measures diastolic function, fluid status, and ventricular dyssynchrony • Identifies vegetations of valves • Visualizes structures at the back of the heart, such as the left atrial appendage
Chest radiography (x-ray)	71020	$300	• Shows heart, lungs, airway, blood vessels, and lymph nodes • Shows bones of your spine and chest, including breastbone, ribs, collarbone, and the upper part of spine • Chest x-ray is the most common imaging test or x-ray used to find pathology Negative chest x-ray: Normal results Positive chest x-ray: Infection, consolidation, fluid

(continued)

Examination	Procedure Code	Cost	Results
EKG	93000	$500 to $1200	• Quick and noninvasive procedure • Records the electrical impulse produced by every heartbeat to gain information about a patient's heart, such as duration of heart contraction, the direction of the impulse, and the strenght of the contraction
Doppler ultrasound	93970–93971	Average is $230	• Noninvasive test that can be used to measure vessel blood flow and blood pressure through high-frequency sound waves • Can estimate how fast blood flows by measuring the rate of change in its pitch (frequency) • This test may be done as an alternative to more-invasive procedures, such as arteriography and venography, which involve injecting dye into the blood vessels so that they show up clearly on x-ray images • A Doppler ultrasound test may also help check for trauma/injury to veins and arteries
Complete blood count (CBC)	85025	$75	The CBC typically has several parameters that are created usually from an automated cell counter White blood count (WBC) • Indicates is the number of white blood cells • High WBC can be a sign of infection, and in association with unilateral leg edema, warmth and fever might be associated with a local cellulitis • WBC is also increased in certain types of leukemia • Low WBC can be a sign of bone marrow diseases or an enlarged spleen • Low WBC is also found in HIV infection in some cases (*Editor's note*: The vast majority of low WBCs in our population are not HIV related) Hemoglobin (Hgb) and hematocrit (Hct) • Hgb is the amount of oxygen-carrying protein contained within the red blood cells (RBCs) • Hct is the percentage of the blood volume occupied by RBCs • In most laboratories, Hgb is actually measured, whereas Hct is computed using the RBC measurement and the mean corpuscular volume (MCV) measurement • Purists prefer to use the Hgb measurement as it is more reliable; low Hgb or Hct suggests anemia • Anemia can be due to nutritional deficiencies, blood loss, destruction of blood cells internally, or failure to produce blood in the bone marrow • High Hgb can occur due to lung disease, living at high altitudes, or excessive bone marrow production of blood cells

Examination	Procedure Code	Cost	Results
Complete blood count (CBC) (*continued*)			MCV • This helps diagnose a cause of an anemia. Low values suggest iron deficiency; high values suggest deficiencies of either vitamin B_{12} or folate, ineffective production in the bone marrow, or recent blood loss with replacement by newer (and larger) cells from the bone marrow Platelet count (PLT) • This is the number of cells that plug up holes in your blood vessels and prevent bleeding • High values can occur with bleeding, cigarette smoking, or excess production by the bone marrow • Low values can occur from premature destruction states, such as immune thrombocytopenia, acute blood loss, drug effects (such as heparin), infections with sepsis, entrapment of platelets in an enlarged spleen, or bone marrow failure from diseases such as myelofibrosis or leukemia • Low platelets also can occur from clumping of the platelets in a lavender-colored tube • You may need to repeat the test with a green-top tube in that case

CLINICAL DECISION MAKING

Case Study Analysis

The advanced practice nurse performs the assessment and physical examination on the patient and finds the following data: Vital signs 156/102, 88 HR, 36.9t, oxygen concentration 96. Without jugular venous pressure (JVP) distension at 30 degrees, heart sounds reveal distant S3 gallop, breath sounds equal with faint crackles bilaterally in bases, rate 18 to 20 and unlabored at rest. Abdomen exam is soft without rebound, guarding, no distension of fluid shift, and skin is without spider angioma. Patient with notable bilateral pitting edema to below knee with somewhat obscured ankle landmarks. Without warmth/tenderness or drainage to suggest cellulitis. Without unilateral edema, calf, or thigh discomfort. No history of coagulopathies and no previous history of pulmonary embolism or deep vein thrombosis. Without known renal disease or cancers. CBC shows normal white blood count, which is reassuring. No anemia, no thrombocytopenia, renal profile shows no electrolyte disturbance or significant acidosis. Comprehensive metabolic panel shows blood glucose normal, normal protein/normal liver function tests, and normal electrolytes. Brain natriuretic peptide (BNP) returns 242 suggestive of early heart failure; troponin 0.0; urinalysis without signs of infection, cocasts, and no hematuria. EKG in a normal sinus rhythm of 88, without ST segment elevation or depression. There is poor precordial R wave progression, and low limb lead voltage. Also notable is high precordial QRS voltage. Chest x-ray shows slight bilateral blunting of costophrenic angles, suggestive of fluid. No appreciable consolidation or effusion.

Diagnosis: Early congestive heart failure

FURTHER READING

Burkhoff, D., Mauer, M., & Packer, M. (2003). Heart failure with a normal ejection fraction: Is it really a disorder of diastolic function? *Circulation, 107,* 656–658.

Ha, J., Lulic, F., Bailey, K., Pellikka, P. A., Seward, J. B., Tajik, A. J., & Oh, J. K. (2003). Effects of treadmill exercise on mitral inflow and annular velocities in healthy adults. *American Journal of Cardiology, 91,* 114–115.

Hunt, S. A., Abraham, W. T., Chin, M. H., Feldman, A. M., Francis, G. S., Ganiats, T. G., . . . Yancy, C. W.; American College of Cardiology Foundation; American Heart Association. (2009). 2009 Focused update incorporated into the ACC/AHA 2005 guidelines for the diagnosis and management of heart failure in adults: A report of the American College of Cardiology Foundation /American Heart Association Task Force on practice guidelines developed in collaboration with the International Society for Heart and Lung Transplantation. *Journal of American College of Cardiology, 53*(15), e1–e90.

Jessup, M., Abraham, W. T., Casey, D. E., Feldman, A. M., Francis, G. S., Ganiats, T. G., . . . Yancy, C. W. (2009). 2009 focused update: ACCF/AHA guidelines for the diagnosis and management of heart failure in adults: A report of the American College of Cardiology Foundation/American Heart Association task force on practice guidelines developed in collaboration with the International Society for Heart and Lung Transplantation. *Journal of American College of Cardiology, 53*(15), 1343–1382.

Lubien, E., DeMaria, A., Krishnaswamy, P., Clopton, P., Koon, J., Kazanegra, R., . . . Maisel, A. S. (2002). Utility of B-natriuretic peptide in detecting diastolic dysfunction: Comparison with Doppler velocity recordings. *Circulation, 105*(5), 595–601.

Mauer, M., Spevack, D., Burkhoff, D., & Kronzon, I. (2004). Diastolic dysfunction: Can it be diagnosed by Doppler echocardiography? *Journal of American College of Cardiology, 44,* 1543–1549.

Morrison, L. K., Harrison, A., Krishnaswamy, P., Kazanegra, R., Clopton, P., & Maisel, A. (2002). Utility of a rapid B-natriuretic peptide assay in differentiating congestive heart failure from lung disease in patients presenting with dyspnea. *Journal of American College of Cardiology, 39*(2), 202–229.

Mueller, C., Scholer, A., Laule-Kilian, K., Martina, B., Schindler, C., Buser, P., . . . Perruchoud, A. P. (2004). Use of B-type natriuretic peptide in the evaluation and management of acute dyspnea. *New England Journal of Medicine, 350*(7), 647–654.

Wells, P. S., Anderson, D. R., Bormanis, J., Guy, F., Mitchell, M., Gray, L., . . . Lewandowski, B. (1997). Value of assessment of pretest probability of deep-vein thrombosis in clinical management. *Lancet, 350*(9094), 1795–1798.

Wells, P. S., Anderson, D. R., Rodger, M., Ginsberg, J. S., Kearon, C., Gent, M., Turpie, A. G., Bormanis, J., . . . Hirsh, J. (2000). Derivation of a simple clinical model to categorize patients probability of pulmonary embolism: Increasing the models utility with the SimpliRED D-dimer. *Journal of Thrombosis and Haemostasis, 83*(3), 416–420.

MOUTH LESIONS

Case Presentation: *A 16-year-old Caucasian female tells you she has multiple mouth lesions. According to the patient, she had been experiencing these painful mouth lesions over the past several weeks with increasing severity.*

INTRODUCTION TO COMPLAINT

- Ulcer that occurs on the mucous membrane of the oral cavity
- Usually an open lesion in the mouth
- Very common occurrence due to association with many diseases and imbalances
- Often causes pain and discomfort
- May alter patient's nutritional state

Different conditions can cause mouth sores, including:

- **Aphthous ulcer (canker sores)** appears white or yellow in the middle, and red around the edges and are caused by certain foods, infections, and biting the tongue or inside of the cheek.
- **Oral thrush** is caused by *Candida albicans*. Presents as whitish plaques in the mouth and can vary from painless to mild soreness.
- **Mouth cancer** appears on the lips or tongue. Mouth cancer can also cause the inside of the mouth, lips, or tongue to turn pale or dark in color. Symptoms are not painful and are discovered only after a routine medical or dental exam.
- **Leukoplakia** is white or gray patches inside the mouth or on the tongue. Patches can be thick and usually develop over time due to irritations the inside of the mouth. Smoking and chewing tobacco are examples of these irritants.
- **Herpetic mucositis** is caused by the herpes simplex virus (HSV) type 1. It is ulcerative and usually presents in multiple spots in the mouth.
- **Acute necrotizing stomatitis** is caused by bacterial infections in the immune-deficient patient. Presenting symptoms include pain, fever, necrotic, or bloody ulcers.
- **Cheilitis** lips appear "chapped" and get red and scaly. Causes include windburn, licking the lips a lot, and certain medicines and foods. Two types exist: *Actinic cheilitis* is caused by too much sun and can later turn into lip cancer. *Angular cheilitis* is caused by a bacterial infection, and usually occurs in older people whose dentures don't fit well. Cheilitis causes redness and cracking in the corners of the mouth.

- **Mucositis** is inflammation of the mucosal surfaces throughout the body and typically involves redness and ulcerative sores in the soft tissues of the mucosa. Oral mucositis manifests as erythema, inflammation, ulceration, and hemorrhage in the mouth and throat.

HISTORY OF COMPLAINT

Symptomatology

Ask about the following characteristics of each symptom using open-ended questions:

- Onset (sudden or gradual)
- Chronology
- Current situation (improving or deteriorating)
- Location
- Radiation
- Quality
- Timing (frequency, duration)
- Severity
- Precipitating and aggravating factors
- Relieving factors
- Associated symptoms
- Effects on daily activities
- Previous diagnosis of similar episodes
- Previous treatments
- Efficacy of previous treatments

Directed Questions to Ask

- How long has it been present?
- Does it come and go?
- Have you had any oral or dental procedure done lately?
- Any food triggers?
- Reaction to drugs?
- Stress level lately?
- Where is the location?
- Any other sores in the body?
- Is it single or in multiples?
- How big or how small?
- Is it increasing or decreasing in size?
- What is the color?
- Is it soft or hard?
- Does it bleed?
- What precipitates bleeding?
- Is it painful?
- What is the pain rating 0 to 10?
- What precipitates and aggravates the pain?
- What relieves the pain?
- Does it affect eating, swallowing, or taste?
- Do you know anyone who has had the same symptom?
- Any associated symptoms? Fevers? Malaise? Fatigue? Swollen nodes?
- Does it affect your daily activities?

- Have you been seen by a practitioner before for the same complaint?
- What was the diagnosis?
- What treatments were used?
- Did treatment relieve the sores?

Assessment: Cardinal Signs and Symptoms

- Mouth and throat
- Dental status
- Bleeding
- Discharge
- Presence of sores anywhere else
- Sore throat
- Aching tooth and gums
- Dysphagia
- Neck
- Swollen lymph nodes
- Pain
- Swelling
- Associated symptoms
- Fever
- Malaise
- Fatigue

Medical History: General

- Medical and surgical history
- Allergies
- List of all medication
- Herbal and traditional medication

Medical History: Specific to Complaint

- Frequents mouth sores
- Dental procedures
- Site of sore related to new denture or procedure
- Intake of food than precipitate mouth sores

PHYSICAL EXAMINATION
Vital Signs

- Temperature
- Pulse
- Respirations
- SpO_2 (oxygen saturation)
- Blood pressure (BP)

General Appearance

- Apparent state of health
- Appearance of comfort or distress
- Color
- Nutritional status
- State of hydration

- Hygiene
- Match between appearance and stated age

Mouth and Throat Inspection
- Lips: color, lesions, symmetry
- Oral cavity: breath odor, color, lesions of buccal mucosa
- Teeth and gums: redness, swelling, caries, bleeding
- Tongue: color, texture, lesions, tenderness of floor of mouth
- Throat and pharynx: color, exudates, uvula, tonsillar symmetry, and enlargement

Neck Inspection
- Symmetry
- Swelling
- Masses
- Active range of motion
- Thyroid enlargement

Palpation
- Tenderness, enlargement, mobility, contour, and consistency of nodes and masses
- Nodes: pre and postauricular, occipital, tonsillar, submandibular, submental, anterior and posterior cervical, supraclavicular
- Thyroid: size, consistency, contour, position, tenderness

CASE STUDY
History

Question	Response
Was the onset sudden or gradual?	It was sudden
Do you have any fever?	Yes, it was 101 this morning
Do you have any aches?	Yes, I am very achy
Is it hard to swallow?	Yes, it is so painful
Are you able to drink fluids?	Yes, I am drinking some fluids, but it hurts
If 10 is the worst pain you have ever had, what number is this pain	9 or 10
Do you have a headache?	Mild headache here (points to front of head)
Do you have a rash?	No
Do you have fatigue?	Yes, I am so tired
Do you have nasal congestion?	No, I'm not stuffy
Do you have a cough?	No, I'm not coughing
Do you have vomiting?	No, my stomach is okay
Have you been exposed to anyone who has sore throat or strep?	No, not that I know of

Physical Examination Findings

- VITAL SIGNS: temperature 100.4°F; pulse 82, regular; respirations 20; SpO_2 99%; BP 128/88
- GENERAL APPEARANCE: anxious, uncomfortable, skin flushed, good skin turgor, unable to eat, can drink cool liquids and eat ice/popsicles, reports 3 lb weight loss, not sleeping
- MOUTH AND THROAT: lips clear, oral cavity; buccal mucosa with four lesions, two on upper palate, one under tongue, and one patient described "lie bump" on top of tongue all with yellow centers, red, edematous, and painful; no geographic tongue, halitosis
- NECK: tracheal symmetry, good range of motion
- PALPATION: submental and submandibular lymph nodes soft, tender, and free moving bilaterally

DIFFERENTIAL DIAGNOSIS

Differential Diagnosis	Aphthous Ulcer	HSV	Oral Cancer
Onset	Abrupt	Abrupt	Gradual
Painful	Yes	Yes	No
Fever	Low	Either	No
Red halo	Yes	No	Either
White/yellow center	Yes	No	No
Vesicles	No	Yes	No
Nodes	Either	No	No

DIAGNOSTIC EXAMINATIONS

Examinations	Procedure Code	Cost	Results
Complete blood count (CBC) with differential	85025	$75	• Search for low white blood cells (WBCs): can be a sign of bone marrow disease or enlarged spleen • Agranulocytosis: failure of the bone marrow to produce enough neutrophils to fight infection • This causes an overgrowth of yeast, and can cause bacterial and viral infections • Neutropenia
Viral culture and polymerase chain reaction (PCR) tests	87252	$75	• Herpes simplex can be the cause of oral lesions • A positive viral culture can mean that the patient has been exposed to the virus • A negative result suggests absence of infection with HSV

CLINICAL DECISION MAKING
Case Study Analysis

- Lesions were in the upper palate, under tongue, presenting with yellow centers, redness, swelling along with pain followed by halitosis.
- Presents with a low-grade temperature of 100.8°F, CBC was slightly elevated, +1 soft, mobile but tender submandibular and submental node, which suggests an inflammatory response.

Diagnosis: Aphthous ulcer (canker sores)

FURTHER READING

Murchison, D. F. (2012). *Recurrent aphthous stomatitis.* Retrieved from http://www.merckmanuals .com/professional/dental_disorders/symptoms_of_dental_and_oral_disorders/recurrent _aphthous_stomatitis.html

Rhoads, J., & Petersen, S. (2013). *Advanced health assessment and diagnostic reasoning* (2nd ed.). Sudbury, MA: Jones & Bartlett.

NECK PAIN

Case Presentation: A 42-year-old construction worker presents to an urgent care clinic complaining of acute neck pain for 3 days.

INTRODUCTION TO COMPLAINT

Neck pain can be acute or chronic and can significantly disrupt activities of daily living (ADL).

Acute Pain

- Trauma (whiplash, strain, fracture)
- Overuse (strain)
- Infection (meningitis, lymphadenopathy from infection)
- Cardiac (angina)
- Systemic disease

Chronic Pain

- History of trauma
- Structural deformity
- Thoracic outlet syndrome
- Neuropraxia (peripheral nerve injury)
  - Entrapment of nerve (carpal tunnel syndrome [CTS])
  - Overuse syndrome
- Systemic disease

HISTORY OF COMPLAINT

Symptomatology

Ask about the following characteristics of each symptom using open-ended questions:

- Systemic disease (hypertension [HTN], cardiac disease, diabetes mellitus, osteoporosis)
- Surgical history
- Allergies (medication and seasonal)
- Medications currently used: daily and as needed (prescription, birth control pill [BCP] and over-the-counter [OTC] drugs, including herbal and traditional therapies)
- Previous neck injury, trauma
- Severity of complaint
- Precipitating and aggravating factors
- Relieving factors
- Associated symptoms
- Effects on daily activities

- History of neck pain
- Previous diagnosis of similar episode:
  - When
  - Frequency
- Previous treatments
  - Efficacy of previous treatments
- Was imaging done?
  - Findings

Directed Questions to Ask

Acute Neck Pain

- Was the onset sudden or gradual?
- What were you doing when it started?
- Was there any trauma prior to onset?
- What is your level of pain on a scale of 0 to 10?
  - When is the pain worse?
  - What makes the pain worse?
  - Does the pain keep you awake at night/awaken you from sleep?
- Does pain radiate to upper extremities?
- Describe the pain
- Do you have any associated chest pain or dyspnea?
- Do you have associated shoulder pain?
- Any recent upper respiratory symptoms? (lymphadenopathy)
- Do you have pain with range of motion (ROM)?
  - Is ROM limited?
- Is there associated upper extremity weakness?
  - Describe distribution of weakness
  - Is it constant or intermittent? (If intermittent, describe what precipitates the pain)
- Do you have a headache (HA)?
  - Describe HA and where it is? Whole head, back of neck, right, or left?
- Do you have peripheral paresthesias (numbness, tingling)?
  - Where and what side? That is, the right fourth and fifth digits? Bilateral hands?
- Do you have dizziness or visual changes?
- Do you have fever or sign of infection?
  - Have you been exposed to anyone with meningitis?

Chronic Neck Pain

- Previous diagnosis of similar episode:
  - When?
  - Frequency (are episodes increasing)?
- Previous treatments
  - Efficacy of previous treatments
- Was imaging done?
  - Findings
- Is this episode similar?
- What were you doing when it started?
- Was there any trauma prior to onset?
- What is your level of pain on a scale of 0 to 10?
  - When is the pain worse?
  - What makes pain worse?
  - Does the pain keep you awake at night/awaken you from sleep?
- Do you have pain with ROM?
  - Is ROM limited?

- Is there associated upper extremity weakness?
  - Describe distribution of weakness
  - Is it constant or intermittent? (If intermittent, describe what precipitates the pain)
- Do you have a headache?
  - Describe HA and where it is? Whole head, back of neck, right, or left?
- Do you have peripheral paresthesias (numbness, tingling)?
  - Where and what side? That is, the right fourth and fifth digits? Bilateral hands?
- Do you have dizziness or visual changes?

Assessment: Cardinal Signs and Symptoms

Head, Scalp, Eyes, Ears, Nose, Throat
- Upper respiratory symptoms
- Scalp and dental status (recent infections)
- Visual changes
- Lesions (herpes zoster)

Shoulders
- Shoulder pain
- History of shoulder trauma: recent or remote
- Pain with ROM
- Lesions (herpes zoster)

Chest
- Chest pain
- Shortness of breath
- Lesions? (herpes zoster)

Back
- Thoracic or lumbar pain
- Pain with ROM
- Lesions? (herpes zoster)

Other Associated Symptoms
- Fever
- Fatigue
- Dizziness

Medical History: General

- History: negative for systemic illness, cardiac disease, HTN, diabetes mellitus, previous neck pain/trauma/injury
- Past surgery: negative

Medical History: Specific to Complaint

- Medications: currently using OTC ibuprofen 400 mg two to three times per day without relief
- Allergy: NKDA (no known drug allergies)

PHYSICAL EXAMINATION
Vital Signs

- Temperature
- Pulse

- Respiration
- Blood pressure
- SpO_2 (oxygen saturation)

General Appearance

- Apparent state of health
- Appearance of comfort or distress
- Color and temperature of skin
- Nutritional status
- State of hydration
- Hygiene
- Match between appearance and stated age
- Difficulty with gait or balance

Head, Eyes, Ears, Nose, Throat (HEENT)

- General HEENT examination to rule out infection that may be causing lymphadenopathy

Neck

- Inspect
  - Position patient is holding head, neck, shoulders
  - Symmetry of neck and thyroid
    - Swelling
    - Visible spasm or mass
  - Compare sternocleidomastoid, trapezius, anterior and posterior triangles for symmetry
  - Presence of jugular venous distention
- Palpate
  - Bony tenderness: neck and shoulder
    - If localized cervical bony tenderness with history of trauma, *stop examination*, apply hard cervical collar, and get imaging as soon as possible
  - Localized muscle spasm and symmetry neck and shoulder
    - Sternocleidomastoid, trapezius, anterior and posterior triangles
    - Localized muscle tenderness neck and shoulder
    - Thyroid
    - Cervical lymph nodes: occipital, pre- and postauricular, tonsillar, submaxillary, submental, superficial, and deep cervical chain anterior/posterior, infra- and supraclavicular
- Evaluate ROM of neck (after it has been determined there is no bony tenderness and cervical fracture has been ruled out). Observe for evidence of pain with ROM and if symmetrical right to left
  - Flexion
  - Extension
  - Rotation
  - Lateral flexion
- Evaluate ROM of shoulders. Observe for evidence of pain with ROM and if symmetrical right to left:
  - Abduction
  - Adduction
  - Internal and external rotation
- Evaluate distal neurological status if complaints of paresthesia

CASE STUDY
History

Question	Response
Was the onset sudden or gradual?	*Began 1 hour after motor vehicle accident (MVA) 3 days ago*
What were you doing when it started?	*Was driving car home*
Was there any trauma prior to onset?	*Minor MVA (rear-ended, low speed), did not hit head*
What is your level of pain on a scale of 1 to 10?	*Initially, 2 to 3 on 10, today 8/10*
When is the pain worse?	*At work (construction worker)*
What makes pain worse?	*Moving neck in any position*
Describe pain	*Feels very tight at back of neck and left upper back*
Does pain radiate to upper extremities	*No, just in back of neck*
Does the pain keep you awake at night/ awaken you from sleep?	*Yes, interfering with sleep*
Do you have any associated chest pain or dyspnea?	*No*
Do you have associated shoulder pain?	*No*
Any recent upper respiratory symptoms? (lymphadenopathy)	*No*
Do you have pain with ROM?	*Yes, with all movement*
Is ROM limited?	*Yes*
Is there associated upper extremity weakness?	*Not that I know of*
Do you have a headache?	*Yes, worse in the morning*
Describe HA and where it is?	*Back of neck, top of head*
Do you have peripheral paresthesias (numbness, tingling)?	*No, my hands are okay*
Do you have dizziness or visual changes?	*No visual change/dizziness*
Do you have a fever or sign of infection?	*I feel okay other than my neck*

Physical Examination Findings

- VITAL SIGNS: temperature 98.8°F; respiratory rate (RR) 16; heart rate (HR) 108, regular; BP 142/84
- GENERAL APPEARANCE: well developed, appropriate for age; looks uncomfortable
- HEENT: no tenderness to palpation or evidence of upper respiratory infection

- NECK:
  - Holding head/neck to right with visible left trapezius spasm
  - No cervical bony tenderness to palpation
  - Left upper trapezius with palpable spasm and tenderness left of midline at base of neck
  - No cervical lymphadenopathy
  - Thyroid examination symmetrical, no tenderness or enlargement
  - Decreased and painful neck ROM with all movement
  - Full ROM of shoulder but complains of pain in neck with movements
  - Negative meningeal signs
- CHEST: lungs are clear in all fields; heart S1 S2 no murmur, gallop, or rub
- SKIN: no rashes
- EXTREMITIES: normal gait, sensation intact distal digits

DIFFERENTIAL DIAGNOSIS

Differential Diagnosis	Neck Strain	Cervical Disc Displacement	Cervical Fracture	Meningitis
Pain	+	+ or −	+	−
Headache	+ or −	+ or −	+ or −	+
Decreased ROM	+	−	+	+
Paresthesias	−	+	+	−
Vision disturbances	−	−	−	+
Fever	−	−	−	+

DIAGNOSTIC EXAMINATION

Examination	Procedure Code	Cost	Results
Physical examination of the neck	92511	$100 to $200	Evaluation of nose, nasopharynx, pharynx, and larynx Normal examination
CT scan: neck	70492	$1000 to $5000	Visualized neck structures ruling out hematomas, fractures, soft tissue trauma Negative for fractures
Lumbar puncture	62270	$3000 to $5000	To test for bacterial meningitis • Lumbar puncture tests collect spinal fluid from around the brain and spinal cord and analyze protein levels, glucose levels, cell counts, and the presence of infectious organisms Alerts for: • Cloudy spinal cord fluid • High spinal cord pressure • An increase in fluid antibodies • Abnormal glucose levels • Increased white blood cells (WBCs) • Bacterial markers in fluid

CLINICAL DECISION MAKING

Case Study Analysis

The APN performs the history and physical examination on the patient and finds the following pertinent positives and negatives.

The pertinent positives are:

- History of low-speed rear-ended MVA likely causing neck to move forward/backward
- Pain started about 1 hour after accident and has progressively worsened
- Describes pain as tightness that is worse in the morning
- Visible left trapezius spasm
- Tender to palpation
- Decreased and painful ROM of neck

The pertinent negatives are:

- Did not hit head and did not have neck pain at time of the accident
- No pain at the time of injury
- No radiating pain or paresthesias
- Normal vital signs
- No evidence of acute infection (negative HEENT examination)
- No lymphadenopathy
- No cervical bony tenderness

Diagnosis: *Cervical strain*

FURTHER READING

Family Practice Notebook. (2011). *Chronic neck pain.* Retrieved October 5, 2013, from http://www.fpnotebook.com/Ortho/Sx/ChrncNckPn.htm

Meredith, P. V., & Moran, N. M. (2000). *Adult primary care* (pp. 608–610). Philadelphia, PA: W.B. Saunders Company.

Seidel, H. M., Ball, J. W., Dains, J. E., Flynn, J. A., Solomon, B. S., & Stewart, R. W. (2011). *Mosby's guide to physical examination* (7th ed.). St Louis, MO: Mosby Elsevier.

PAINFUL INTERCOURSE

Case Presentation: A 24-year-old female complained of painful intercourse. She states she has been experiencing painful intercourse for the past 6 months.

INTRODUCTION TO COMPLAINT

- Recurrent or persistent genital pain that occurs just before, during, or after vaginal intercourse.
- Causes include structural or physical causes, psychological or emotional factors.

Physical Causes

- Insufficient lubrication
  - Insufficient foreplay
  - A drop in estrogen level (after childbirth, during breastfeeding)
  - medication (antidepressants, blood pressure [BP] medications, sedatives, some antihistamines, and certain birth control pills)
- Injury, trauma
  - Traumatic injury to pelvis or peritoneum
  - Pelvic surgeries
  - Female circumcision
  - Episiotomy scars
  - Congenital abnormality.
- Inflammation, infection, or skin disorders
  - Infection in the genital area or urinary tract
  - Eczema or other skin problems
- Certain illnesses or conditions
  - Endometriosis
  - Pelvic inflammatory disease
  - Uterine fibrosis
  - Retroverted uterus
  - Ovarian cysts
  - Cystitis
  - Uterine prolapse
  - Irritable bowel syndrome
- Surgical or medical treatments
  - Scarring from surgeries that involve the pelvic area
  - Hysterectomy, radiation, or chemotherapy for cancer treatments

Emotional Causes

- Psychological problems, such as anxiety, depression concerns about physical appearance, fear of intimacy, or relationship
- Stress tightens pelvic floor muscles making intercourse painful
- History of sexual abuse

HISTORY OF COMPLAINT

Symptomatology

Ask about the following characteristics of each symptom using open-ended questions:

- Systemic disease (hypertension [HTN], cardiac disease, diabetes mellitus, osteoporosis)
- Surgical history
- Medications currently used: daily and as needed (prescription, birth control pill [BCP], and over-the-counter [OTC] drugs, including herbal and traditional therapies)
- Previous trauma
- Severity of complaint
- Precipitating and aggravating factors
- Relieving factors
- Associated symptoms
- Effects on daily activities

Directed Questions to Ask

- Do you have any sensation of burning?
- What are the circumstances that you think contributed to the painful intercourse?
- Do you have any redness or swelling?
- Do you have any lower abdominal pain?
- Do you have itching?
- Do you have any irritation or abrasions?
- Do you have any lesions?
- Do you have any warty growths?
- Do you have any dryness?
- Did you notice any unusual profuse discharge or malodorous discharge?
- Do you have any bleeding during or after intercourse?
- Do you have any voluntary or involuntary contraction of muscles around the vagina?
- Where are your injuries?

Assessment: Cardinal Signs and Symptoms

Vagina
- Sensation of burning
- Redness or swelling
- Lower abdominal pain
- Itching
- Irritation or abrasions
- Lesions
- Warty growths

- Dryness
- Presence of unusual profuse discharge or malodorous discharge
- Bleeding
- Voluntary or involuntary contraction of muscles around the vagina
- Where are your injuries?

Cervix
- Lower abdominal pain
- Foul smelling discharge
- Tenderness inside vagina

Other Associated Symptoms
- Fever
- Unusual fatigue
- Abdominal pain
- Rectal pain

Medical History: General
- Have you had any stomach or gastric problems in the past?
- Have you had any surgeries in the past? I had episiotomies from my deliveries.
- Are you allergic to anything like medication, food, or plants?
- Do you currently use any medications which include any prescription medications?
- Do you use any over the counter medications?
- Did you use any herbal preparations or traditional therapies? Vitamins?

Medical History: Specific to Gynecology
- When did you have your first menses? How old were you?
- When was your last menstrual period? Are they regular?
- Do you use tampons? Do you douche?
- Have you had a Pap smear? If so, when was it last done?
- When was the last time you had vaginal intercourse?
- Do you use contraceptives?
- Have you ever been pregnant? How many pregnancies?
- What are the outcomes of your pregnancies?
- Have you had any abortions?
- Do you have any history of infections like gonorrhea, syphilis, or herpes?

PHYSICAL EXAMINATION
Vital Signs
- Temperature
- Pulse
- Respiration
- BP
- O_2 saturation

General Appearance
- SKIN: note the condition of skin and observe for bruising or other signs of physical trauma
- ABDOMEN: palpate all four quadrants

- PELVIC: external genitalia visualization; observe for bruises, lesions, swelling, lacerations
- INTERNAL EXAMINATION: on speculum examination, observe for condition and color of vaginal mucosa; signs of inflammation, ulcers, and tears; observe color and position of the cervix, ulceration, nodules, cysts, or injury; observe the shape of the cervix and particularly for bleeding or discharge and, if present, its color, consistency, and odor
- BIMANUAL EXAMINATION: palpate for nodules or tenderness in the vagina, including the region of the urethra and bladder; palpate the cervix and note mobility and presence of tenderness; palpate the ovaries and note any pain on palpation
- RECTOVAGINAL EXAMINATION: during the rectovaginal exam, palpate for tenderness; palpate the uterus, and right and left adnexa for nodularity or thickening
- RECTAL EXAMINATION: observe and palpate the rectum for hemorrhoids, anal fissures, or other abnormalities

CASE STUDY

History

Question	Response
Do you have a history of any medical conditions like diabetes, high blood pressure, or high cholesterol?	*No*
Have you had any heart problems or history of cardiovascular disease?	*No*
Do you have any breathing or respiratory problems?	*No*
Have you had any stomach or gastric problems in the past?	*No*
Have you had any surgeries in the past?	*I had episiotomies from my deliveries*
Are you allergic to anything like medication, food, or plants?	*No*
Do you have any history of infections like gonorrhea, syphilis, or herpes?	*I had a yeast infection once but never anything else*
Do you currently use any medications, which includes any prescription medications?	*I take birth control pills, Tylenol for pain, and Alka-Seltzer for nausea*
Do you use any over the counter medications?	*Yes, what I just told you*
Do you use any herbal preparations or traditional therapies?	*Vitamins*
When did you have your first menses?	*When I was 12 years old*
How is your menstruation?	*I am regular*
When was your last menstrual period (LMP)?	*2 weeks ago*

Question	Response
When was your last sexual activity?	*Last night*
Do you use contraceptives, tampons, or douches?	*I use birth control pills, tampons, but no douches*
Have you ever been pregnant? How many pregnancies?	*Two*
What are the outcomes of your pregnancies?	*Two healthy little girls*
Have you had any abortions?	*No*
How many living children?	*Two*
When was your last Pap smear test?	*One year ago*
Do you have any redness or swelling?	*Yes*
Do you have any sensation of burning?	*No*
Can you tell me about your pain?	*I have pain in my vagina. It happened when my husband forced me to have sexual intercourse when I didn't want to.*
Is it a sudden pain or gradual pain?	*Sudden pain*
Where is the pain? Is it near the outside, occurring at the start of the intercourse, or do you feel it farther in, when your partner is pushing deeper?	*The pain is in my vagina and it started when he shoved into me.*
Does it radiate to your pelvis, hips or any part of your abdomen?	*No*
On a scale of 0 to 10 with 0 no pain and 10 the worst pain you ever had, how do you rate your pain?	*10*
When does the pain start? How long does the pain last? Does it hurt only during intercourse? Did this pain start only 6 months ago?	*The pain started when he forced himself into me! He doesn't give me time to adjust to his size. Yes, the pain has existed every time we have sex.*
What are the circumstances that you think contributed to the painful intercourse?	*When he forces me to have sex and I am not ready*
Does your husband get angry with you when you complain of painful intercourse?	*Yes, he gets angry*
Is there anything that makes it worse?	*When he drinks he is abusive. There is no talking to him.*
Is there some other discomfort that accompanies the painful intercourse?	*My legs hurt, my bottom hurts, and I can feel my insides shaking around*

Question	Response
How does this pain affect your daily activities?	*I feel angry and sad*
Did you try to treat this pain with medications or other remedies?	*I take Tylenol*
How effective was the treatment or remedies?	*It helps*
Do you have any redness or swelling?	*Yes*
Do you have any lower abdominal pain?	*No*
Do you have itching?	*No*
Do you have any irritation or abrasions?	*Yes*
Do you have any lesions?	*No*
Do you have any warty growths?	*No*
Do you have any dryness?	*Yes*
Did you notice any unusual profuse discharge or malodorous discharge?	*No*
Do you have any bleeding?	*Afterward*
Do you have any voluntary or involuntary contraction of muscles around the vagina?	*Don't know what you mean? I feel tight and shaky*
Where are your injuries?	*I have bruises on my legs, and down there*

Physical Examination Findings

- VITAL SIGNS: Temperature 98.7°F (oral), pulse 72 beats/min, respiration 18 breaths/min, BP 120/72 mmHg
- GENERAL APPEARANCE:
  - Well-developed healthy looking 24-year-old muscular female
  - Admitted due to injuries sustained when her husband hit her
  - Complaints of dyspareunia during sexual intercourse
  - In good state of health and presently is not in distress
  - Height: 5 feet 6 inches tall
  - Weight 122 pounds
  - Well groomed in tight jeans and blouse with heavy makeup but appears clean
  - Appearance matches with her age
  - Mood looks sad and depressed
  - Skin clear without bruising, lesions, pale
  - Nutritional status is good
  - No difficulty with gait or balance
- THE SKIN:
  - Warm
  - Dry
  - No open lesions

- Color of the skin looks pale but no rashes, scarring, or warts
- Many bruises with finger imprints were noted on the inner aspect of thighs bilaterally, abdomen, and buttocks
- PELVIC EXAMINATION:
  - External genitalia examination: bruises noted on the labia majora and labia minora. But no lesions, swelling or ulcerations noted; no obvious signs of rectocele or cystocele
  - Internal examination: on speculum examination, vaginal mucosa looks very dry, color pink, moist, no signs of inflammation, or ulcers; tear in vaginal orifice is noted; color and position of the cervix are normal, no ulceration, nodules, cysts or injury; the shape of the cervix is slit-like, with no lesions noted; no bleeding or discharges evident within normal parameters
  - Bimanual examination: no nodularity or tenderness in the vagina, including the region of the urethra and bladder; palpation of the cervix was normal and mobile with no tenderness; head of the uterus was smooth and nontender; ovaries were mobile and no pain was evident upon exam
  - Rectovaginal examination: rectovaginal examination was normal and nontender; uterus, right and left adenexa appear within normal limits; no nodularity or thickening of the uterosacral ligaments were noted
  - Rectal examination: rectal examination revealed no abnormalities; no hemorrhoids, anal fissures were observed

DIFFERENTIAL DIAGNOSIS

Differential Diagnosis	Insufficient Lubrication	Atrophic Vaginitis	Pelvic Inflammatory Disease	Sexually Transmitted Diseases	Endometriosis
Onset	Sudden, during insertion of penis	Well-defined coitus pain	During sex	During sex	During/ after sex and menstruation
Quality of pain	Deep, during/after intercourse, rated 10/10	Difficulty and severe pain with penetration	Severe	Severe	Deep pelvic pain
Tenderness	+	+	+	+	+
Discharge	−	−	Severe	+	+ or −
Itching	−	+	+	+	−
Burning	+	+	+	+	+
Abrasion	++	+	−	+	−
Bruises	++	−	−	−	−

(continued)

Differential Diagnosis	Insufficient Lubrication	Atrophic Vaginitis	Pelvic Inflammatory Disease	Sexually Transmitted Diseases	Endometriosis
Dryness/friction	Severe	Severe	–	–	+ or –
Erythema	+	+	+	+	–
Irritation/rawness	+	+	–	–	–
Lesions	–	–	+	+	–
Abnormal bleeding	Spotting	+ or –	Excessive	+	+
Fever	–	–	+	+	+
Palpable mass	–	–	+	–	+

DIAGNOSTIC EXAMINATION

Pelvic Examination	Procedure Code	Cost	Results
External genitalia examination	88147	$150	• Vulva and labia: erythema, excoriations, and induration • Bruises noted on the labia majora and labia minora • Swelling/redness and abrasions
Internal vaginal examination	88141 to 88158	$150	• Using speculum: Can identify the presence of any foreign body like tampons, condom, etc., injury, or vaginal infections • Vaginal walls look dry with no lubrication • Can identify any pelvic dysfunctions • Can find any lesion or mass • Cotton swab test or Q tip test during a pelvic exam to diagnose provoked vestibulodynia (vestibulititis; PVD)
Vaginal rectal examination	88141 to 88158	Part of office visit cost	• To determine pelvic/uterine dysfunctions • Identify pelvic mass • Identify retroverted uterus
Bimanual examination	88141 to 88158	Part of office visit cost	• Assess the status of uterus, fallopian tube, and cervical motion tenderness

(*continued*)

Pelvic Examination	Procedure Code	Cost	Results
Laboratory diagnostic studies	88150 to 88155	$55 to $75	• Urine test for pregnancy is the first laboratory test • Test for pH > 4.5 is consistent with bacterial vaginitis or atrophic vaginitis • Potassium hydroxide and wet mount preparation will show any bacterial vaginitis (clue cells) and yeast infection • Urine analysis and culture: Microscopic examination can rule out cystitis or pelvic inflammatory disease (PID) • Serology for screening syphilis, e.g., VDRL • Blood test for complete blood count and erythrocyte sedimentation rate (ESR) to check the infection
Pap smear	88150 to 88155	$35	• Send sample for culture (results can show any infection, sexually transmitted infections [STIs], PID)
Pelvic ultrasound or pelvic x-ray	76870	$525	• Determine pelvic organ dysfunction, injury and whether ectopic pregnancy • Identify presence of retroverted uterus

CLINICAL DECISION MAKING

Case Study Analysis

Results of pelvic exam (PE) and diagnostic study on a 24-year-old female reveal the diagnosis of insufficient lubrication of vagina. Evidence to support this is based on complaints of painful intercourse with dryness, friction, burning, tearing, and irritation. The physical examination reveals abrasions, bruises, and a tear. Diagnostic tests included urine pregnancy test, Pap smear, and pelvic ultrasound and pelvic x-ray.

> *Diagnosis:* Vaginal trauma due to insufficient lubrication because of inadequate arousal before sexual intercourse

FURTHER READING

Dains, B., & Scheibel, P. (2007). *Advanced health assessment and clinical diagnosis in primary care* (3rd ed.). St. Louis, MO: Mosby/Elsevier,

Heim, L. J. (2001). Evaluation and differential diagnosis of dyspareunia. *American Family Physician*, 63(8), 1535–1545.

Mayo Clinic. (n.d.) *Painful intercourse (dyspareunia).* Retrieved from http://www.mayoclinic.com/health/painful-intercourse/DS01044

Rhoads, J., & Petersen, S. (2013). *Advanced health assessment and diagnostic reasoning* (2nd ed.). Sudbury, MA: Jones & Bartlett.

RUNNY NOSE

Case Presentation: *A 30-year-old computer programmer presents to your clinic complaining of a 12-day history of a runny nose.*

INTRODUCTION TO COMPLAINT

- Rhinorrhea (nasal discharge) is a common complaint in family practice.
- The most frequent etiologies include common viral upper respiratory infections, acute bacterial rhinosinusitis, allergic rhinitis, and nonallergic rhinitis.

Acute Viral Rhinosinusitis

- The most common upper respiratory viruses causing the "common cold" are rhinoviruses (30%–50%), coronaviruses (10%–15%), and other viruses (5%).
- Symptoms typically start with a sore throat which then progresses to include nasal congestion, rhinorrhea, sneezing, cough, and mild malaise.
- If there is a fever, it tends to resolve after 24 to 48 hours.
- Nasal purulence which is defined as nasal discharge with color can occur with a viral respiratory rhinitis, particularly in the later stages of the illness.

Acute Bacterial Rhinosinusitis

- It is a complication of a viral upper respiratory infection (URI) in only 0.5% to 2% of cases
- Symptoms of acute viral rhinosinusitis (AVRS) and acute bacterial rhinosinusitis (ABRS) are similar
- During the first 10 days, many cases of acute ABRS resolve spontaneously
- Both ABRS and AVRS can produce purulent nasal discharge
- Consider bacterial sinusitis if there is unilateral sinus pain or maxillary tooth pain that tends to worsen when bending over
- Another sign of ABRS is seen when a presumed viral URI initially improves and then worsens after 5 to 6 days ("double sickening")
- If symptoms are severe, including fever > 39°C or 102°F with purulent nasal discharge and a headache for 3 or more days, this is consistent with ABRS that requires consideration of immediate antibiotic treatment
- Red-flag symptoms requiring emergent referral include persistent high fever, meningeal signs, or visual disturbances

Allergic Rhinitis

- Affects 10% to 30% of adults in the United States
- Common symptoms include rhinorrhea, sneezing, nasal pruritus, and congestion
- Frequently accompanied by conjunctivitis symptoms, such as increased lacrimation, irritation, and pruritus of the eyes

- Can appear seasonally in which case it is usually associated with outdoor allergens, which are primarily pollens
- Perennial allergic rhinitis is more frequently caused by indoor allergens, such as dust mites, mold spores, pet dander, and cockroaches
- Objective findings in allergic rhinitis can include a pale and boggy nasal mucosa, watery rhinorrhea, and injected conjunctiva
- Patients can develop dark circles under the eyes, called allergic shiners, secondary to nasal congestion
- A nasal crease is also a common finding caused by patients pushing up on the tip of the nose ("allergic salute") in an attempt to relieve nasal pruritus

Nonallergic Rhinitis

- Fifty percent of patients presenting with rhinitis may have either nonallergic rhinitis or a combination of nonallergic and allergic rhinitis, which is termed "mixed rhinitis."
- Symptoms of nonallergic rhinitis as compared to allergic rhinitis more frequently include nasal congestion, postnasal drainage, and later age of onset (> 20 years).
- Conjunctivitis symptoms are not present.
- Tends to be exacerbated by weather changes and irritant odors.
- Except in the mixed variety, it is associated with negative allergen testing by either an immunoassay blood test or skin testing.

HISTORY OF COMPLAINT

Symptomatology

Ask about the following characteristics of each symptom using open-ended questions:

- Onset
- Duration, timing, frequency
- Character of the discharge, color
- Location of discharge, from nose only or also in throat
- Pain in the sinus areas
  - What makes it worse?
  - What makes it better?
- Treatments or medications

Directed Questions to Ask

Head, Eyes, Ears, Nose, Throat (HEENT)
- Do your ears hurt or feel congested? Does your face hurt? If so, where is the pain? What would you rate the pain on a scale of 0 to 10?
- Do you have a headache? If you do, rate the pain on a scale of 0 to 10.
- Is your nose congested?
- Do you have a runny nose? If so, what color is it?
- Does your nose itch?
- Does your throat hurt?
- Do your upper teeth hurt?
- Do the glands in your neck seem swollen or painful?
- Does any nasal drainage drip down into your throat?
- Have you had any change in your vision?
- Do you have a stiff neck?
- Are your eyes bothering you?

Respiratory
- Are you coughing?
- If so, are you coughing up any phlegm?
- If the patient has a cough productive of sputum, inquire as to the quantity, color, and whether there is any hemoptysis. It also can be helpful to ask the patient whether the sputum seems to be coming from the nose/throat (postnasal drainage) versus the chest.
- Are you wheezing?
- Do you feel short of breath?

Gastrointestinal
- Have you had any stomach symptoms, such as nausea, vomiting, or diarrhea?
- Are you taking any medication? Are you allergic to any medications?
- Do your symptoms seem to be improving, staying the same or getting worse?

Assessment: Cardinal Signs and Symptoms
- Runny nose
- Sinus pressure
- Headache
- Dizziness

Medical History: General
- Past medical history
- Past surgical history
- Current medications
- Allergies to medications
- Social history
- Family history

Medical History: Specific to Complaint
- Sinus infection
- History of allergies
- Nasal or sinus surgery
- Exposure to anyone with similar symptoms

PHYSICAL EXAMINATION
Vital Signs
- Any signs of acute distress?
- Does the voice sound normal or do you hear signs of nasal congestion and/or hoarseness?
- Any obvious difficulty breathing, such as mouth breathing, wheezing, or increased respiratory effort?

General Appearance
Ears
- Are the ear canals normal?
- Are the tympanic membranes normal?

Eyes
- Has there been any change in your vision?
- Are your eyes bothering you?
- Are your eyes itchy?

Nose
- Is there mucosal swelling? Is it unilateral or bilateral?
- What is the color of the mucosa, such as pale, red, or normal?
- Is there any drainage? If so, what color is it?

Throat
- Is there any redness?
- Is there any exudate?
- If the tonsils are present, are they enlarged?
- Is there any postnasal drainage?
- Is there a cobblestone appearance to the posterior pharynx?

Neck
- Is there any submental, submandibular, tonsillar, anterior, or posterior cervical adenopathy?
- Test for nuchal rigidity by having the patient touch her chin to her chest. If she is able to there is no nuchal rigidity or meningeal signs.

Lungs
- Are the lungs clear bilaterally?
- Is there good air exchange?
- Is she breathing easily?

Heart
- Is there a regular rate and rhythm?
- Is there a murmur or abnormal heart sounds?

Skin
- Is there a rash?

CASE STUDY
History

Question	Response
When did your symptoms begin?	*They began 12 days ago*
Do your symptoms seem to be improving, staying the same, or getting worse?	*At first, it seemed like I just had a cold, which after 5 or 6 days seemed to be improving. Then, I suddenly felt worse.*
How much do your symptoms affect you?	*I am so tired that it is difficult for me to work*
Have you been able to work or exercise?	*I stayed home yesterday and today. I have not gone to the gym since my symptoms got worse. I do not seem to have the energy.*
Does anything seem to make your symptoms better or worse?	*When I lean over, my face becomes more painful, especially on the right side*

Question	Response
Have you tried any medications or home remedies for your symptoms?	*I tried using my Neti pot. It makes my nose feel a little better for a short time.*
Are your symptoms worse at a certain time of day, when you are indoors vs. outdoors or in any certain positions, such as supine versus standing?	*When I am lying flat at night, I cough more*
Have you had a fever, chills or fatigue?	*I may have had a fever the past few days*
Have you ever had similar symptoms?	*Yes, I did about 3 years ago*
Have you ever been diagnosed with a sinus infection?	*Yes, when I had similar symptoms 3 years ago*
Do you have a history of allergies?	*Yes, I tend to get a runny nose during the spring-time pollen season. However, this time of year (winter), my allergies are not a problem.*
Do your ears hurt or feel congested?	*Initially, they felt a little full. Now, they are feeling better.*
Does your face hurt? If so, where would you rate the pain on a scale of 0 to 10?	*Yes, my cheekbones and forehead hurt, particularly on the right side. I would rate the pain as 5/10.*
Do you have a headache?	*Only my forehead and cheeks hurt*
Is your nose congested?	*Yes, it feels very congested*
Do you have a runny nose? If so, what color is the drainage?	*Yes, I have a runny nose. The drainage varies between clear and yellow. It particularly tends to be yellow on the right side.*
Does your nose itch?	*No, it does not*
Does your throat hurt?	*It feels irritated*
Do your upper teeth hurt?	*Yes, they are mildly painful*
Do the glands in your neck seem swollen or painful?	*They are a little tender*
Does any nasal drainage drip down into your throat?	*Yes, it particularly bothers me at night when I am lying flat*
Has there been any change in your vision?	*No, my vision is normal*
Are your eyes bothering you?	*My eyes are fine*
Is your neck stiff?	*No, it feels normal*
Are you coughing?	*Sometimes, the drainage in my throat causes me to cough, particularly when I lie down*
If so, are you coughing up any phlegm?	*Yes, occasionally I am*

Question	*Response*
Do you have a cough productive of sputum and, if so, what is the quantity, color, and is there hemoptysis. Also, does the sputum seem to be coming from the nose/throat [postnasal drainage] or the chest?	*It is a small amount of yellowish phlegm, which seems to be coming from the back of my throat*
Are you wheezing?	*No, I am not*
Do you feel short of breath?	*No, I do not*
Have you had any stomach symptoms, such as nausea, vomiting or diarrhea?	*No, my stomach is fine*

Physical Examination Findings

- VITAL SIGNS: Blood pressure (BP) 110/70, pulse (P) 88, respiratory rate (RR) 16, temperature (T) 100.4°F (38°C), O_2 saturation 99% on room air
- GENERAL APPEARANCE: No signs of acute distress. Patient appears mildly fatigued. She is breathing through her mouth. Voice has a nasal quality to it.
- EARS: Ear canals: normal
- TYMPANIC MEMBRANES: Normal
- EYES: Conjunctiva: no injection, no increase in lacrimation or purulent drainage
- NOSE: Bilateral erythema and edema of turbinates with significant yellow drainage on the right. Nares: Obstructed air passages
- THROAT: Posterior pharynx: mildly injected, scant postnasal drainage (PND), no exudate, tonsils 1+, no cobblestoning (common in allergic disease secondary to enlargement of lymphoid tissue)
- NECK: Anterior cervical lymph nodes: tender but not enlarged. No posterior cervical chain or submental lymph node enlargement or tenderness. Easily touches chin to her chest (no nuchal rigidity).
- LUNGS: Breathing easily. Clear to auscultation bilaterally with good aeration
- HEART: Regular rate and rhythm, no murmur, S3, or S4

DIFFERENTIAL DIAGNOSIS

Symptoms and Signs	Acute Viral Rhinosinusitis	Acute Bacterial Rhinosinusitis	Allergic Rhinitis	Nonallergic Rhinitis
Fever	< 24–48 hours	*> 48 hours	Afebrile	Afebrile
Purulent drainage	+ or −	+ (often unilateral)	Usually clear	Usually clear
Congestion	+	+	+ or −	+
Nasal pruritus	Negative	Negative	Positive	+ or −

Symptoms and Signs	Acute Viral Rhinosinusitis	Acute Bacterial Rhinosinusitis	Allergic Rhinitis	Nonallergic Rhinitis
Postnasal drainage	+ or −	+	+ or −	+ or −
Duration until symptom improvement	< 10 days	> = 10 days	Seasonal vs. perennial	Perennial
Triggers	None	None	Allergens	**Nonallergic
Sinus pain	If present: bilateral	Unilateral and worse with bending over	If present: bilateral	None
***Nasal mucosa	Red, swollen turbinates, purulent drainage less common, if present is bilateral	Red with purulent drainage, which is often unilateral	Pale/boggy	Possibly boggy
Eye symptoms	Possible increased lacrimation	None	Frequently increased lacrimation and pruritus	Absent
Nasal pruritus	Absent	Absent	Frequently present	+ or −

*Bacterial sinusitis can also present without fever; temp > = 39°C with severe symptoms, consider immediate antibiotic treatment.
**Examples of common triggers are weather changes (cold), spicy or hot food, scents.
***Typical appearance with frequent exceptions.

DIAGNOSTIC EXAMINATIONS

Viral URI versus acute bacterial sinusitis: Differentiating ABS versus AVS is primarily a clinical diagnosis. Currently, there is no diagnostic testing in the primary care setting that has a high sensitivity and specificity. Both sinus x-rays and computed tomography (CT) scans can have false positives. They can show air/fluid levels and mucosal thickening of the sinuses in both viral and bacterial sinusitis. Forty two percent of sinus CT scans show abnormalities in healthy sample populations. Furthermore, sinus CT scans are associated with significant radiation exposure.

Allergy testing is not routinely done for differentiating ABS versus AVS. In more chronic conditions, if underlying allergies are suspected, allergy testing can be done. Skin testing is the most accurate and least expensive diagnostic available. Immunoassay tests (a blood test) can also be performed. Their highest sensitivity is for airborne allergens. However, they are less accurate than skin tests and more costly. Nurse practitioners may choose to use immunoassay tests if skin testing is not readily available, patients prefer a blood draw to a visit with a specialist, or if patients are not able or willing to stop antihistamine use prior to skin testing.

Test Name	Current Procedural Terminology (CPT)	Cost	Description
Immunoglobulin E (IgE) level	82785	Approximately $100	An elevated IgE is not a sensitive marker for allergic rhinitis. A level of >100 is present in only 44% of patients with allergic rhinitis.
Allergen-specific immunoassay tests	Varies depending on which test is ordered. Geographically appropriate panels of tests are frequently available. An example would be the Northwest Allergen Panel, which tests for common allergens in the Pacific Northwest.	Approximately $200 to $800 depending on the number of tests ordered.	Tests for the presence of IgE to specific allergens, such as dust or ragweed. The specificity is < 100% as can have positive allergen-specific IgE with no associated allergic symptoms on exposure. Therefore, if there is a positive result for a specific allergen, it is important to correlate it with the patient's symptoms before diagnosing this specific allergen as the cause of the patient's symptoms.

CLINICAL DECISION MAKING

Case Study Analysis

Through a thorough history and physical the advanced practice nurse has found the following pertinent positives:

- The patient has had a "double sickening" with what likely began as AVRS, which then progressed to ABRS
- She has unilateral sinus pain
- She has purulent nasal discharge
- Her upper teeth are painful
- She has increased sinus pain when she bends over
- She has a history of seasonal allergies
- She is not taking any medications, nor does she have any allergies to medications

Pertinent negatives: Does not have symptoms typical of a more allergic presentation, such as nasal pruritus, clear watery rhinorrhea, or conjunctival symptoms

> *Diagnosis: Although your patient does have a history of seasonal allergic rhinitis, you determine that your patient's current symptoms and physical exam are consistent with a diagnosis of acute bacterial rhinosinusitus.*

FURTHER READING

Williamson, I. G., Rumsby, K., Benge, S., Moore, M., Smith, P. W., Cross,. M, & Little, P. (2007). Antibiotics and topical nasal steroid for treatment of acute maxillary sinusitis: A randomized controlled trial. *Journal of the American Medical Association, 298*(21), 2487–2496. doi:10.1001/jama.298.21.2487

SHORTNESS OF BREATH

Case Presentation: *A 50-year-old Caucasian female presents to your clinic with a complaint of shortness of breath for the past 3 days.*

INTRODUCTION TO COMPLAINT

- Shortness of breath (SOB) otherwise known as "dyspnea" is the subjective feeling of an uncomfortable sensation of breathing discomfort and labored breathing.
- It is common, usually occurs as a result of cardiac or respiratory function disorders, may represent conditions from psychiatric to nonurgent to life threatening, and can be acute or chronic.
- Immediate attention is necessary to determine whether the cause is life threatening and to address the airway, breathing, and circulation and stabilize prior to further evaluation and treatment.

Life-Threatening Causes

Upper Airway
- Tracheal foreign objects (food, coins, bones, dentures, pills)—uncommon in adults
- Angioedema—swelling of the lips, tongue, posterior pharynx, larynx over days to hours; causes are allergic, nonsteroidal anti-inflammatory drugs (NSAIDs), or angiotensin-converting enzyme (ACE)-inhibitor induced
- Anaphylaxis—severe swelling of upper airway, tongue; triggered by allergens; progresses to airway occlusion over a period of a few minutes to hours
- Infections of the pharynx and neck cause swelling and pain (epiglottitis, peritonsillar abscess, retropharyngeal abscess)
- Airway trauma/burns—hemorrhage and swelling

Pulmonary
- PULMONARY EMBOLISM: Dyspnea at rest, tachypnea, pleuritic chest pain; history of deep vein thrombosis; prolonged bed rest due to illness, surgery (orthopedic), trauma; prolonged sitting after a long car, bus, train, or airplane trip; women who are pregnant, postpartum, or taking oral contraceptives; smoking; bleeding abnormalities causing blood to be hypercoagulable; obstruction of pulmonary arterial vasculature usually from an embolus (clot) from deep venous system of lower extremities; may occur from a clot in upper extremities; may present as acute or chronic
- PNEUMOTHORAX: Trauma; spontaneous, can happen to anyone

Cardiac
- ACUTE CORONARY SYNDROME (STEMI/NONSTEMI, UNSTABLE ANGINA): Dyspnea may be the only presentation in females, elderly, and diabetics; caused by the lack of blood supply to a coronary artery by inflammation within the vessel walls and/or clot; ± history of coronary artery disease.

- CARDIAC ARRHYTHMIA: Dyspnea can be a result of cardiac conduction abnormalities (atrial flutter, atrial fibrillation, heart block, tachyarrhythmias); may be due to myocardial ischemia.
- CARDIAC TAMPONADE: Acute dyspnea; classic triad of hypotension, distended neck veins, and muffled heart tomes may be absent; and causes are trauma, malignancy, drugs, infection.

Causes of Acute Dyspnea

Chronic Obstructive Pulmonary Disease Exacerbation
- Viral
- Bacterial infection
- Inadequate medication management
- Can be chronic
- Consider pulmonary embolism (PE) if the patient does not improve with chronic obstructive pulmonary disease (COPD) treatment

Asthma Exacerbation
- Dyspnea with wheezing
- Severe if using accessory muscles, diaphoresis, fragmented speech, fatigue
- Viral
- Allergens
- Exercise
- Bacterial infection
- Environmental precipitants
- Inadequate medication management
- Can be chronic

Lung Infections
- Productive cough, fever, pleuritic chest pain
- Not acute unless underlying COPD or asthma
- Bronchitis
- Pneumonia

Congestive Heart Failure (CHF)
- New onset (acute) or chronic
- Dyspnea on exertion (DOE), orthopnea, paroxysmal nocturnal dyspnea (PND), and cough to severe pulmonary edema
- Tachypnea, pulmonary crackles, + jugular vein distension (JVD), S3 gallop, peripheral edema
- Can follow myocardial ischemia and arrhythmia
- Pump failure (systolic or diastolic)
- Volume overload

Valvular Dysfunction
- Dyspnea may be a symptom of aortic stenosis or mitral regurgitation

Severe Anemia
- Dyspnea due to lack of oxygen-carrying capacity
- Acute (hemorrhage) or chronic

Anxiety
- Dyspnea, chest pain, palpitations, dizziness with anxiety
- Underlying anxiety or depression
- Diagnosis of exclusion as common with other medical conditions

Viral Infections
- Caused by a viral illness, such as the common cold, the most common type of viral illness (mild)

HISTORY OF COMPLAINT
Symptomatology

Ask about the following characteristics of each symptom using open-ended questions:

- Onset (sudden, gradual, or chronic)
- Character
- Duration
- Current situation (improving or deteriorating)
- Pain and location
- Quality
- Radiation
- Severity
- Timing (onset, frequency, duration)
- Exacerbating and relieving factors
- Medication usage
- Associated symptoms
- Effects on daily activities
- Previous diagnosis of similar episodes
- Previous treatments
- Efficacy of previous treatments

Directed Questions to Ask

- Was the onset sudden or gradual?
- Can you describe it?
- How long has this been going on?
- Have you had any recent trauma or falls?
- On a scale of 0 to 10 how bad is it?
- What seemed to trigger it?
- Is it getting better or worse?
- What makes it worse?
- What have you tried to relieve it?
- Has this ever happened before?
- What has worked in the past to relieve it?
- Do you have asthma, COPD, hypertension (HTN), heart disease, or diabetes?
- What medications are you on?
- Have you been taking your medications?
- Do you have a cough?
- If yes to cough, is it dry and hacking or productive?
- If dry and hacking are you wheezing?
- If productive what color is the sputum?
- Has the sputum changed in color?
- Is the SOB worse after coughing?
- Is the SOB worse with lying down?
- Is the SOB worse with exertion?
- How far can you walk before SOB? Is this worse than before?

- How many stairs can you climb before SOB? Is this worsening?
- Does the SOB awaken you at night?
- What relieves the SOB?
- Do you have any fevers or chills?
- Do you have any body aches?
- Do you have nausea, vomiting, or diaphoresis?
- Does your chest hurt?
- Have you had chest pain before?
- Is this like chest pain you have had before?
- If yes, point to where your chest hurts and does it radiate?
- On a scale of 0 to 10 rate your chest pain.
- Describe your chest pain—is it sharp, stabbing, one side, or dull and aching, with a heaviness?
- Is your chest pain worse with deep breaths?
- Is your chest pain worse with movement?
- Does it hurt to touch your chest?
- Does your arm, shoulder, back, or neck hurt?
- What makes your chest pain worse or better?
- Do you have weakness?
- Do you have palpitations, dizziness, or syncope?
- Do you have fatigue?
- Do you smoke?
- Have you had any recent surgeries or travel?
- Have you ever had a blood clot before?
- Could you be pregnant?
- Does one side hurt worse than the other?
- Do you use cocaine?
- Are you under a great deal of stress?

Assessment: Cardinal Signs and Symptoms

Ask about the presence of the following:

Head, Eye, Ear, Nose, Throat (HEENT)
- Headache
- Sinus congestion
- Postnasal drip
- Dental status
- Oral lesions
- Sore throat
- Dysphagia

Neck
- Pain
- Swelling
- Enlarged glands

Respiratory
- Productive cough
- Chest tightness
- Wheezing
- Unilateral leg swelling
- Environmental exposure
- History of intubation

Cardiac
- Chest pain
- Pink, frothy sputum
- Extremity swelling
- Orthopnea, DOE

Gastroenterology
- Nausea and vomiting

Psychiatric
- Stress
- Medication overdose

Neurology
- Headaches
- Trauma

Other Associated Symptoms
- Fever
- Malaise
- Weakness
- Fatigue

Medical History: General
- Medical conditions and surgeries
- Allergies (seasonal as well as others)
- Medications currently used (inhalers, antihypertensive medications, birth control pills [BCPs], antibiotics, diuretics, pain medications and over-the-counter [OTC] drugs)
- Herbal preparations and traditional therapies

Medical History: Specific to Complaint
- Asthma
- COPD
- Cardiac history
- Surgeries
- Pregnancy
- Smoker

PHYSICAL EXAMINATION
Vital Signs
- Temperature
- Pulse
- Respiration
- Pulse oximetry
- Blood pressure (BP)

General Appearance
- Apparent state of health
- Appearance of comfort or distress
- Color
- Nutritional status

- State of hydration
- Hygiene
- Match between appearance and stated age
- Difficulty with gait or balance

HEENT
- HEAD: trauma, tenderness to palpation
- EYES: conjunctiva and sclera, pupils, equal, round, and reactive to light and accommodation (PERRLA), extraocular muscles (EOMs)
- NOSE: discharge at nares, inflammation, turbinates, discharge/congestion
- FACE: facial swelling, maxillary/frontal tenderness
- THROAT: airway obstruction
- LIPS: color, lesions, symmetry, swelling
- TONGUE: color, texture, lesions, tenderness of floor of mouth, swelling
- THROAT AND PHARYNX: color, exudates, uvula, tonsillar symmetry, and enlargement

Neck
- Symmetry, swelling, masses
- Active range of motion
- Thyroid enlargement
- JVD
- Trachea midline

Palpation
- Tenderness, enlargement, mobility, contour, and consistency of nodes and masses
- Nodes—pre- and postauricular, occipital, tonsillar, submandibular, submental, anterior and posterior cervical, supraclavicular
- Thyroid: size, consistency, contour, position, tenderness

Lungs
- INSPECTION: intercostal, subcostal, and supraclavicular retractions; abnormalities of chest wall with inspiration/expiration; prolongation of expiratory phase; rash or tenderness
- AUSCULTATION: equal breath sounds, wheezes, rhonchi, rales
- PALPATION: tenderness
- PERCUSSION: dullness secondary to effusion or consolidation; hyperresonance of a pneumothorax

Cardiovascular
- Auscultation: size, rhythm, gallops, murmurs, clicks, or rubs
- JVD
- Extremities for edema

Gastroenterology
- Bowel tones
- Tenderness
- Masses or organomegaly

Vascular
- Femoral and extremity pulses
- Capillary refill
- Clubbing, edema, calf tenderness or swelling, erythema
- Unilateral lower extremity swelling

CASE STUDY
History

Question	Response
Was the onset sudden or gradual?	*It came on gradually over 3 days*
Can you describe it?	*I feel like I can't get enough air*
How long has this been going on?	*3 days*
Have you had any recent trauma or falls?	*No*
On a scale of 0 to 10 how bad is it?	*About a 6*
What seemed to trigger it?	*My kids are sick with colds*
Is it getting better or worse?	*Worse, that's why I came in*
What makes it worse?	*Coughing*
What have you tried to relieve it?	*My inhaler—but it's not working anymore. I think it's empty.*
Has this ever happened before?	*Yes, always after a cold*
What has worked in the past to relieve it?	*My inhaler and steroids*
Do you have asthma, COPD, HTN, heart disease, or diabetes?	*Asthma*
Have you ever been intubated?	*No*
Have you ever been to the emergency room for your asthma?	*No, I come to the clinic*
What medications are you on?	*Albuterol*
Have you been taking your medications?	*Yes, too much and it ran out last night. It didn't help anyway*
Do you have a peak flow meter at home?	*I can't find it*
Do you have a cough?	*Yes, hacking and wheezing all the time*
If yes to cough, is it dry and hacking or productive?	*Yes*
If dry and hacking, are you wheezing?	*Yes*
If productive, what color is the sputum?	*No sputum*
Has the sputum changed in color? Is the SOB worse after coughing?	*Yes—I cough so hard I vomit*
Is the SOB worse with lying down?	*Yes, my nose is plugged and worse in the morning*
Is the SOB worse with exertion?	*I've been home resting*
How far can you walk before SOB? Is this worse than before?	*I cough with any walking*

Question	*Response*
How many stairs can you climb before SOB? Is this worsening?	*Yes*
Does the SOB awaken you at night?	*Yes, it did last night*
What relieves the SOB?	*Not coughing*
Do you have any fevers or chills?	*Yes, mild*
Do you have any body aches?	*Yes*
Do you have nausea, vomiting, or diaphoresis?	*Vomit after coughing*
Does your chest hurt?	*Yes, from coughing*
Have you had chest pain before?	*My chest gets sore from coughing. Same as before.*
Is this like chest pain you have had before?	*Yes*
If yes, point to where your chest hurts and does it radiate?	*My chest is sore all across the top from coughing*
On a scale of 0 to 10 rate your chest pain.	6
Describe your chest pain—is it sharp, stabbing, one side, or dull?	*It is sore from coughing*
Do you feel a heaviness?	*No*
Is your chest pain worse with deep breaths?	*Yes—I can't take a deep breath or I cough*
Is your chest pain worse with movement?	*No*
Does it hurt to touch your chest?	*Yes, across the top*
Does your arm, shoulder, back, or neck hurt?	*No*
What makes your chest pain worse or better?	*Not coughing*
Do you have weakness?	*No*
Do you have palpitations, dizziness, or syncope?	*No*
Do you have fatigue?	*Yes*
Do you smoke?	*No*
Have you had any recent surgeries or travel?	*No*
Have you ever had a blood clot before?	*No*
Could you be pregnant?	*No*
Does one side hurt worse than the other?	*No*
Do you use cocaine?	*No*
Are you under a great deal of stress?	*No*

Physical Examination Findings

- VITAL SIGNS: 99°F; respiratory rate (RR) 30; heart rate (HR) 110, regular; BP 130/60; pulse oximetry 97%
- GENERAL APPEARANCE: well-developed, healthy appearing female with labored breathing at 30 per minute, leaning forward "tripod" position, sweating, coughing, in moderate distress; color is good; able to speak in short sentences; alert and oriented in time, place, and person
- EYES: no injection, anicteric, PERRLA, extraocular movements intact
- NOSE: nares are patent; no nasal discharge; turbinates not swollen; no congestion
- MOUTH: no oral lesions; teeth and gums in good repair; no swelling
- PHARYNX: pink; tonsils normal without exudate; airway is patent; no stridor; no drooling
- FACE: no facial swelling
- NECK: no neck swelling or tenderness with palpation; neck is supple; no JVD; thyroid is not enlarged; trachea midline
- HEART: regular rhythm, rate; S1 and S2 no murmur, gallop, or rub; capillary refill adequate
- LUNGS: breath sounds are equal and symmetrical throughout; chest with expansion; RR labored; tachypneic at 30; expiratory wheezes present throughout all fields; no rhonchi or bibasilar crackles
- ABDOMEN: soft, nontender without masses or organomegaly
- SKIN: no rashes
- EXTREMITIES: no joint pain or swelling; no calf tenderness/swelling; no ankle edema
- NEUROLOGY: without neurological deficits

DIFFERENTIAL DIAGNOSIS

Differential Diagnosis	CHF	Asthma/ COPD	Pulmonary Embolus (PE)	Acute Coronary Syndrome (ACS)	Pneumonia (PNA)
Onset	Either	Either	Sudden	Either	Gradual
Cough	+ or −	+	−	−	+
Fever	−	+ or −	−	−	+
Chills	−	−	−	−	+
Sweats	−	+ or −	+ or −	+ or −	+ or −
Chest tightness	−	+ or −	+	+ or −	−
Orthopnea	+	+ or −	−	+ or −	−
Wheezing	Either + or −	Common	Not common	Not common	Not common
Pleuritic chest pain	−	−	+	+ or −	−

(continued)

Differential Diagnosis	CHF	Asthma/COPD	Pulmonary Embolus (PE)	Acute Coronary Syndrome (ACS)	Pneumonia (PNA)
Calf pain/swelling	+	−	+ One leg	−	−
Anxiety	+	+	+	+	+
Fatigue	+	+	+	+	+
Malaise	+	−	−	+	+
Weakness	−	−	−	+ or −	−

DIAGNOSTIC EXAMINATION

Examination	Procedure Code	Cost	Indications and Interpretation
EKG	93000	$150	An EKG with dyspnea may reveal: • Ischemia and or infarction (ST segment changes) • Arrhythmias/rhythm abnormalities • Enlarged ventricles • Heart valve abnormalities • Global and regional left ventricular function (normal contraction) • Estimate of the ejection fraction or amount of blood pumped out by each • Ventricular contraction • Identify a mural thrombosis (blood clot in the ventricle wall) • Normal EKG cannot rule out cardiac disease • Compare with previous EKG
Posterior–anterior and lateral chest radiograph	71020	$517	An anterior–posterior and lateral chest x-ray (CXR) will reveal • Acute heart failure (cardiomegaly, interstitial edema, and vascular congestion) • Pneumonia—infiltrate considered "gold standard" (may be nondiagnostic if early and/or dehydrated) • Pneumothorax • Pleural effusion • COPD/asthma—large lung volumes and flattened diaphragm suggest air trapping; however, CXR may be normal. • Foreign body—consider with unilateral air trapping • Compare with previous CXR
Cardiac biomarkers (troponin I)	84484	$11	• Cardiac troponin I is specific for cardiac tissue and is detected in the serum only if myocardial injury has occurred • Diagnostic level for increased cardiac risk with the new assay is troponin I > 0.25 ng/mL. A level of 0.1 to 0.25 ng/mL is considered intermediate. A level of < 0.1 ng/mL is considered negative.

Examination	Procedure Code	Cost	Indications and Interpretation
			• By 6 hours after symptom onset using troponin I there is a 95% to 99% detection rate of patients who are ultimately shown to have a myocardial infarction • The assay identifies patients who are at higher risk for cardiac events and mortality • Each increase of 1.0 ng/mL in the cardiac troponin I level is associated with an increase in the relative risk of mortality • The troponin I assay allows early identification and stratification of patients with chest pain suggestive of ischemia, allows identification of patients that present 48 hours to 6 days after infarction, and identifies patients with false-positive elevations in CK-MB (such as in rhabdomyolysis) • A negative troponin I assay does not exclude the diagnosis of unstable angina and does not exclude myocardial infarction of less than 6 hours duration • Serial measurements are necessary to rule out acute coronary syndrome • Repeat troponin assay after initial testing in 6 hours • May be elevated with PE, sepsis, pericarditis, myocarditis, warfarin use
BMP (basic metabolic panel)	80048	$119	The BMP typically has several parameters that are created from an automated cell counter. The most relevant are: • Glucose: Energy source for the body; a steady supply must be available for use, and a relatively constant level of glucose must be maintained in the blood (hypoglycemia, hyperglycemia) • Na (sodium): Electrolyte imbalance (hyponatremia, especially in elderly fragile females) • K (potassium): Electrolyte abnormality (hyperkalemia or hypokalemia, especially due to medications or recent illnesses with vomiting and diarrhea) • BUN (blood urea nitrogen): Waste products filtered out of the blood by the kidneys; conditions that affect the kidney have the potential to affect the amount of urea in the blood (dehydration) • Creatinine: Waste product produced in the muscles; filtered out of the blood by the kidneys so blood levels are a good indication of how well the kidneys are working (acute/chronic renal insufficiency)
CBC (complete blood count) with differentials	85025	$75	The CBC typically has several parameters that are created from an automated cell counter. The most relevant are: White blood count (WBC) • The number of white cells • High WBC can be a sign of infection • WBC is also increased in certain types of leukemia

(continued)

Examination	Procedure Code	Cost	Indications and Interpretation
CBC (complete blood count) with differentials (*continued*)			• Low white counts can be a sign of bone marrow diseases or an enlarged spleen • Low WBC is also found in HIV infection in some cases. (Editor's note: The vast majority of low WBC counts in our population is not HIV related.) Hemoglobin (Hgb) and hematocrit (Hct) • Hgb is the amount of oxygen-carrying protein contained within the red blood cells (RBCs) • Hct is the percentage of the blood volume occupied by RBCs • In most labs Hgb is actually measured, whereas the Hct is computed using the RBC measurement and the mean corpuscular volume (MCV) measurement • Purists prefer to use the Hgb measurement as it is more reliable. Low Hgb or Hct suggests an anemia • Anemia can be due to nutritional deficiencies, blood loss, destruction of blood cells internally, or failure to produce blood in the bone marrow • High Hgb can occur due to lung disease, living at high altitudes, or excessive bone marrow production of blood cells MCV • This helps diagnose a cause of anemia. Low values suggest iron deficiency; high values suggest deficiencies of either vitamin B_{12} or folate, ineffective production in the bone marrow, or recent blood loss with replacement by newer (and larger) cells from the bone marrow Platelet count • This is the number of cells that plug up holes in your blood vessels and prevent bleeding • High values can occur with bleeding, cigarette smoking, or excess production by the bone marrow • Low values can occur from premature destruction states, such as immune thrombocytopenia, acute blood loss, drug effects (such as heparin), infections with sepsis, entrapment of platelets in an enlarged spleen, or bone marrow failure from diseases such as myelofibrosis or leukemia • Low platelets also can occur from clumping of the platelets in a lavender-colored tube. You may need to repeat the test with a green-top tube in that case
D-dimer	85379	$20.92	• Use of test depends on patient's pretest probability for PE • Limitations: In patients with low or moderate probability of clots in the deep veins of the leg, a negative D-dimer result generally rules out deep venous thrombosis (DVT). Some patients with blood clots will be false negatives. This is most common among older patients, those who have undergone prolonged hospitalization, and those with markedly elevated C-reactive protein levels.

Examination	Procedure Code	Cost	Indications and Interpretation
			• **Reference range(s)** < 0.50 mcg/mL • **Clinical significance** D-dimer is one of the measurable byproducts of activation of the fibrinolytic system. Quantitation of D-dimer assesses fibrinolytic activation and intravascular thrombosis. D-dimer is of particular value in excluding the diagnosis of venous thromboembolism among patients at high risk.
B-natriuretic peptide (BNP)	83880	$50	• BNP may assist with assessing whether acute decompensaed heart failure is the contributing cause of dyspnea (SOB) • BNP is a hormone that is secreted by the ventricular cells in response to high ventricular filling pressures and is a useful indicator of left ventricular dysfunction • Use caution when interpreting values in patients with chronic heart failure
Peak flow meter with nebulizer treatment	94640	$30	• Peak expiratory flow rate (PEFR) can be useful in differentiating between cardiac and pulmonary causes of dyspnea • Information about presence and severity of airflow obstruction • Determine severity of bronchoconstriction in asthma • Compare to personal best • Assess improvement with nebulizer treatments
Arterial blood gas	82803	$80	• Limited • Oxygenation assessed with transcutaneous pulse oximetry • Provides a more accurate assessment of oxygenation • Provides ability to calculate an alveolar/arterial oxygen gradient • Patients at risk for cardiac or neurologic compromise secondary to hypoxia can be identified • Measures carbon dioxide, which indicates severity of airflow obstruction
Lower extremity duplex venous ultrasound	93971	$100	• Evaluate DVT with high sensitivity (95%) and specificity (95%) for lower extremity DVT • May be a cost-effective first test for evaluating possible PE in patients with signs/symptoms of PE and in those with contraindications to chest CT angiography (CTA; pregnant, renal insufficiency, contrast dye allergy)
Oximetry	94760	$414	• At rest or with exercise is helpful in detecting hypoxia, but not hypercarbia

(*continued*)

Examination	Procedure Code	Cost	Indications and Interpretation
CTA chest	71275	$1000	• Indicated in patients with a high pretest probability of venous thromboembolism, + D-dimer (patients in whom D-dimer is likely to be positive) • Test of choice to rule out PE • CTA will identify a clot as a filling defect in a contrast-enhanced pulmonary artery • Sensitivity 83% to 90% and specificity is 95% • May also be helpful in diagnosis of other problems, such as malignancy, pneumonia, and pulmonary edema)
Ventilation/ perfusion scan (V/Q)	78588	$1200	• Compares emission of radioisotope that is injected into pulmonary arteries with emission of radioisotope that is inhaled into the alveoli • V/Q scan can rule out PE in 96% to 100% of cases when homogenous scintillation is demonstrated through the lung in the perfusion portion • Usefulness is limited as only onethird of V/Q scans will demonstrate findings sufficient to diagnose or rule out PE with certainty • For patients in whom a CTA is contraindicated

CLINICAL DECISION MAKING

Case Study Analysis

The APN performs the assessment and physical examination on the patient and finds the following pertinent positives: gradual onset of worsening dyspnea for 3 days after being exposed to sick children not relieved with inhaler, hacking spasmodic cough with clear sputum, vomit after coughing, RR 30, in moderate distress, unable to speak in full sentences, respirations labored with audible wheezing. Bilateral breath sounds present with end expiratory wheezes. Diagnostic testing reveals peak flows below personal best at 150. Pertinent negatives are absence of fever, pleuritic chest pain, of cough with blood, or purulent sputum. The complete blood count, chemistries, and chest x-ray are normal. The EKG is normal.

Diagnosis: Asthma exacerbation—mild to moderate with viral upper respiratory infection

SHOULDER PAIN

Case Presentation: A 45-year-old male presents to the clinic with right shoulder pain.

INTRODUCTION TO THE COMPLAINT

- Shoulder pain is a very common musculoskeletal complaint. The pain can be intrinsic (in the shoulder joint, tendons, and surrounding ligaments) or referred pain from the neck, chest, or abdomen.
- The shoulder joint is the most complex joint in the human body. Due to this complex network of a number of anatomic structures, the shoulder has tremendous mobility.

Acute Shoulder Pain

- Defined as pain experienced for less than 2 weeks
- Blunt trauma is a common cause of acute shoulder pain. Examples include falls directly on the shoulder, falls onto an outstretched arm.
- Fractures: Clavicle, proximal humerus, and scapula
- Dislocations: 25% of all shoulder injuries; 95% being anterior glenohumeral dislocations
- Younger patients tend to experience sports injuries due to overuse (muscular strain) as well as fractures and dislocations.

Chronic Shoulder Pain

- Involves injury to the rotator cuff. These injuries generally occur in middle age or older patients.
- Rotator cuff injuries result from poor athletic technique, poor muscular conditioning, poor posture, and failure of the subacromial bursa to protect the supporting tendons, which results in an injury from acute inflammation to degenerative thinning and calcification and then finally to a tendon tear.
- Impingement syndrome is used to describe symptoms that occur from the compression of the rotator cuff tendons and the subacromial bursa between the greater tubercle of the humeral head and the lateral edge of the acromion process.
- Older adults tend to present with frozen shoulder (adhesive capsulitis) and symptomatic osteoarthritis.
- Adhesive capsulitis is a stiffened glenohumeral joint that has lost significant range of motion (ROM).
- Any shoulder pain that causes a patient not to use his or her shoulder can lead to decreased mobility and ultimately adhesive capsulitis.
- Osteoarthritis of the glenohumeral joint represents wear and tear of the articular cartilage. It a problem that occurs due to trauma years earlier.
- Osteoarthritis is quite rare and could be due to a secondary cause.

Referred Shoulder Pain

- Generally it is poorly localized or vaguely described.
- Neural impingement at the level of the cervical spine
- Peripheral nerve entrapment distal to the spinal column
- Diaphragmatic irritation due to splenic laceration, perforated viscous, ruptured ectopic pregnancy, intrathoracic tumors, and distension from hepatic capsule can produce ipsilateral pain.
- Myocardial ischemia associated with left shoulder pain

Anatomy of the Shoulder Joint

- This mobility is enhanced by a girdle of three bones, the clavicle, scapula, and proximal humerus.
- There are four articular surfaces (joints): stenoclavicular, acromioclavicular, glenohumeral, and scapulothoracic.
- The glenohumeral joint, commonly called the shoulder joint, is the principal articular surface.
- Intrinsic pain is located in either the glenohumeral structures or the extraglenohumeral structures.
- The glenohumeral structures involved in acute or chronic shoulder pain are the glenohumeral joint and the rotator cuff.
- The rotator cuff is composed of four muscles (supraspinatus, infraspinatus, subscapularis, and teres minor and a cuff around the head of the humerus to which all four muscles attach).
- The glenohumeral ligaments serve as stabilizers, they include the superior, middle, and inferior glenohumeral ligaments.
- Extraglenohumeral structures involved in a shoulder pain complaint are acromioclavicular and sternoclavicular joints and the scapulothoracic articulation.
- Anterior shoulder pain can involve the biceps tendon.
- Three muscles provide additional stability to the glenohumeral joint.
- These muscles include the teres major, latissimus dorsi, and pectoralis major.
- The neural networks of the brachial plexus form proximal to the glenohumeral joint.
- An injury to the brachial plexus can present as shoulder pain.

HISTORY OF COMPLAINT

Symptomatology

Ask about the following characteristics of this symptom (shoulder pain) using open-ended questions:

- Onset (sudden or gradual)
- Chronology
- Current situation (improving or deteriorating)
- Location
- Radiation
- Quality
- Timing (frequency, duration)
- Severity
- Precipitating and aggravating factors
- Relieving factors

- Associated symptoms
- Effects on daily activities
- Previous diagnosis of similar episodes
- Previous treatments
- Efficacy of previous treatments

Directed Questions to Ask

- What is your age?
- Which is your dominant hand?
- What are your work or sports activities?
- Was the onset of shoulder pain sudden or gradual?
- Was there an injury you can recall?
- Describe the injury.
- Can you point to exactly where the pain is?
- Does your shoulder joint feel loose or unstable?
- Do you notice muscle weakness, catching, stiffness?
- What activities were being done at the time of injury? Was the patient lifting overhead, pulling, throwing, or is there no apparent cause for injury or reinjury?
- Does the pain awake the patient from sleep, especially when lying on the affected side?
- Does the pain occur only after activity?
- Does the pain occur during activity but does not restrict performance?
- Does the pain occur during activity and restrict performance?
- Is the pain chronic and unremitting?

Assessment: Cardinal Signs and Symptoms

Neck
- Any neck pain
- Sharp pain radiating from neck to shoulder

Elbow
- Pain
- Decreased ROM

Neurologic (Upper Extremity)
- Numbness
- Paresthesia
- Weakness

Respiratory
- Cough
- Wheezing
- Pleuritic chest pain

Cardiac
- Dyspnea
- Chest pain or discomfort
- Palpitations

Other Associated Symptoms
- Fever
- Night sweats
- Weight loss

Medical History: General

- Past and current medical conditions, especially diabetes (risk factor for "frozen shoulder")
- Previous orthopedic treatments and surgeries
- Any history of prolonged immobility
- Allergies (seasonal as well as others)
- Medication currently used (prescription, birth control pill [BCP], and over-the-counter [OTC] drugs)
- Herbal preparations and traditional therapies

Medical History: Specific to Complaint

- Previous shoulder treatments—diagnostic testing, hospitalizations, surgeries, and pain management

PHYSICAL EXAMINATION

Vital Signs

- Temperature
- Pulse
- Respiration
- SpO$_2$ (oxygen saturation)
- Blood pressure (BP)

General Appearance

- Apparent state of health
- Appearance of comfort or distress
- Color
- Nutritional status
- State of hydration
- Hygiene
- Match between appearance and stated age

Neck
- Swelling
- Tenderness upon palpation
- Active ROM
- *Special test*: Head compression test (with patient sitting on a low stool, stand behind the patient, lock hands together, and then apply gentle but firm downward pressure on head, using both hands locked together)

Elbow
- Swelling
- Tenderness upon palpation
- Active ROM

Shoulder
- INSPECTION: Observe how the patient moves and carries shoulders; inspect front and back of shoulders for any swelling, discoloration, symmetry, muscle atrophy, scars, abrasions, lacerations, and venous distension; observe the height of the shoulders and scapulae.

- PALPATE: Palpate the acromioclavicular joint, sternoclavicular joint, cervical spine, biceps tendon anterior glenohumeral joint, coracoid process, acromion, and scapula; palpate for point tenderness, snapping, grinding and bony crepitus; palpate the area distal and proximal to the pain location.
- ROM: Assess passive and active ROM—forward elevation, abduction, external rotation, internal rotation.
- SPECIAL TESTS: Maneuvers to test for rotator cuff problems—empty can test, Neer's test. Maneuvers to test for acromioclavicular joint disease—cross-arm test. Maneuvers to test for glenohumeral joint stability—apprehension test. Maneuvers to test ROM—scratch test, painful arc test.

Associated Systems for Assessment

A complete assessment of cardiac, respiratory, gastrointestinal, and upper extremity neurology if concerned about referred pain.

- Assess for nerve injury
- Sensation in the arm and hand on the affected side
- Motor function should be evaluated by the major nerves of the extremity
- Assess for arterial blood flow
- Evaluate for circulatory compromise on the affected side
- Capillary refill should be assessed in each finger
- Pulses, radial, ulnar, and brachial, need to be evaluated

CASE STUDY
History

Question	Response
Was the onset sudden or gradual?	It was gradual
How long have you had the pain?	Around 2 weeks or so
Is the pain improving or deteriorating?	Getting worse
Where is the pain located?	Really in the front of my shoulder but does wake me up at night when I roll on my shoulder
What does the pain feel like?	Achy but when I roll on it, it throbs
How often does the pain occur?	When I reach over my head and at night. Otherwise a dull ache that is always there.
How severe is the pain on a scale of 0 to 10?	It is usually about 2 to 3 but with certain movements it can go to a 6 to 7
What aggravates or makes the pain worse?	Overhead movement and rolling on my shoulder at night
What relieves the pain?	I have used muscle rub such as Icy Heat, which helped, putting heat on it. Ibuprofen did not help very much.
Any associated symptoms?	Not really

Question	Response
What effects does this pain have on your daily activities?	*I feel like I am not moving my shoulder as much*
Have you had similar episodes of pain?	*Back in my 20s, I experienced shoulder pain when I was playing basketball*
Do you remember what the diagnosis was of this episode?	*I had some sort of tendonitis but I do not remember the name*
What previous treatments have you tried?	*I think pain killers and rest*
Were the previous treatments effective?	*Yes, it went away*
Directed Questions Related to Shoulder Pain	
What is your age?	*45 years old*
Which is your dominant hand?	*Right hand*
What are your work or sports activities?	*I have been playing more tennis with my wife lately and a couple weekends ago I wallpapered our bathroom*
Was there an injury you can recall?	*No real injury but did hurt a lot worse after our weekend of wallpapering*
Does your shoulder joint feel loose or unstable?	*No*
Do you notice muscle weakness, catching, stiffness?	*Shoulder definitely feels stiff in the morning*
What activities were being done at the time of injury? Was the patient lifting overhead, pulling, throwing, or no apparent cause for injury or reinjury?	*Was playing more tennis as well as wallpapering in the bathroom*
Does the pain awake the patient from sleep, especially when lying on the affected side?	*Rolling over on the affected side does worsen the pain*
Does the pain only occur after activity?	*Pain is worse with overhead lifting, otherwise a general dull ache in shoulder*
Does the pain occur during activity?	*Yes, but does not restrict performance*
Does the pain occur during activity and restrict performance?	*Worried about moving shoulder too much and causing increasing pain*
Is the pain chronic and unremitting?	*Pain is a chronic ache*

Physical Examination Findings

- VITAL SIGNS: 98.71°F; respiratory rate (RR) 16; heart rate (HR) 78, regular; BP 132/80
- GENERAL APPEARANCE: well-developed, healthy-appearing male in no acute distress

- NECK: no tenderness on palpation, full ROM, negative head compression test
- ELBOW: normal appearance bilaterally, no tenderness on palpation, fully active and passive ROM
- SHOULDERS: normal appearance bilaterally, normal strength bilaterally; right shoulder: + tenderness at the subacromium process; normal passive ROM; increased pain with midarc abduction and external pain with impingement testing (Neer and Hawkins's tests), + crepitus noted with abduction greater than 60°
- NEUROLOGICAL: sensation and strength equal bilaterally
- EXTREMITIES PERIPHERAL CIRCULATION: radial, ulnar, and brachial pulses equal bilaterally

DIFFERENTIAL DIAGNOSIS

Differential Diagnosis	ROM	Pain	Loss of Muscle Strength	Numbness
Impingement (tendinopathy, bursitis)	+	+	+	+
Rotator cuff tears	+	+	+	–
Ligament tears	+	+	+	–
Arthritis	–	+	–	–
Gout	–	+	–	–
Glenohumeral joint degenerative joint disease	+	+	+	+

DIAGNOSTIC EXAMINATION

Examination	Procedure Code	Cost	Results
Lidocaine injection test (in office procedure)	96372	? billable	Can be used to confirm the diagnosis of rotator cuff tendonits Can help exclude a diagnosis of frozen shoulder. The point of entry is 1 to 1.5 inches below the midpoint of the acromion The angle of entry parallels the acromion. A 1.5-inch (4 cm) 22-gauge needle is inserted to a depth of 1 to 1.5 inches. And 1 mL of lidocaine is injected into the deltoid and 1 to 2 mL into the subacromial bursa.

(continued)

Examination	Procedure Code	Cost	Results
Shoulder radiograph: complete, minimum of two views	73030	$150 to $200	Overall, radiographic studies are inexpensive, readily available, and easily interpreted. The disadvantages are exposure to radiation, poor tissue, needs radiology technician for high-quality images, two-dimensional view.
			Anterior–posterior and axillary views of shoulder (two views) are necessary to evaluate patients who have experienced trauma, lost ROM, and experience severe trauma
			• Fractures of the proximal humerus, clavicle, and scapula • Glenohumeral dislocations • Glenohumeral osteoarthritis • Acromioclavicular joint arthritis • Sternoclavicular joint arthritis
			Beneficial in osteoarthritis; axillary view demonstrates the joint space narrowing that indicates cartilage destruction
Shoulder MRI without contrast Shoulder MRI with contrast	73221 73222	$1000 to $1500	The advantage of an MRI is its superior contrast resolution; its disadvantages are: it is a costly diagnostic test, it interacts with metals in the body. MRI is the preferred imaging study for patients with suspected impingement and rotator cuff injury. A normal MRI indicates that the likelihood of a rotator cuff tear is less than 10%.
			MRI findings for rotator cuff tears are not highly specific, especially in older patients. The sensitivity and specificity for impingement diagnosis are 93% and 87%, respectively. This diagnostic tool is useful in the evaluation of avascular necrosis, biceps tendinopathy, and rupture.
Ultrasound of shoulder	76881	$150 to $300	The diagnostic accuracy of an ultrasound in the hands of skilled operators is equal to that of an MRI in identifying a number of conditions, including rotator cuff tears, labral tears, biceps tendon tears, and dislocations. It is helpful in detecting complete rotator cuff tears but less helpful in identifying partial tears. Decreased cost and being preferred by a majority of patients are some of the other benefits

CLINICAL DECISION MAKING

Case Study Analysis

The advanced practice nurse performs the assessment and physical examination on the patient and finds the following pertinent positives. Right shoulder pain for 2 weeks due to increase of tennis playing and one weekend of wallpapering. The patient's physical examination notes + tenderness at the subacromium process. Increased pain with midarc abduction and external pain with impingement testing (Neer and Hawkins's tests) + crepitus noted with abduction greater than 60°. Pertinent negatives are absence of trauma, neck pain, and radiation of pain and normal passive ROM.

> **Diagnosis:** *Rotator cuff tendonitis*

SKIN LESION

Case Presentation: *A 70-year-old White retired photographer presents to your clinic with a complaint of a skin lesion.*

INTRODUCTION TO THE COMPLAINT

Skin complaints are some of the most common reasons for seeking care. They can be benign or represent an underlying medical condition. Many skin lesions look similar and so making an accurate diagnosis can be a challenge. Besides a thorough history, assessing the skin in a systematic way is essential to making a diagnosis. Knowing the type of lesion, size, and distribution of the lesion, associated findings, and the patient (child, adult, child starting puberty, elderly, or pregnant female) all aid in sorting out the diagnosis.

HISTORY OF THE COMPLAINT

Symptomatology

Ask about the following characteristics of each symptom using open-ended questions:

- Onset (sudden or gradual)
- Chronology
- Current situation (improving or deteriorating)
- Location
- Radiation
- Quality
- Timing (frequency, duration)
- Severity
- Precipitating and aggravating factors
- Relieving factors
- Associated symptoms
- Effects on daily activities
- Previous diagnosis of similar episodes
- Previous treatments
- Efficacy of previous treatments

Directed Questions to Ask

- Did the lesion start suddenly or come on slowly?
- How long have you had the lesion?
- Do you only have one lesion and where is it located?

- If you have more than one lesion where are they located?
- Can you describe the color, size, and shape of the lesion?
- Is the lesion raised?
- Is the lesion painful?
- Does the lesion have any drainage? Or, is it crusted or scaling?
- Has the appearance of the lesion changed since it appeared?
- Have you had any fevers, chills, itching, fatigue, or decreased appetite?
- Have you ever had a cancer?
- Have you had any recent injury to your skin or trauma?
- Have you traveled recently?
- Have you been exposed to any chemicals in or your home or work?
- Have you been camping, hiking, or working in outdoors?
- Are you taking any medications or drugs?
- Have you started any new medications recently?
- Have you had a change in diet or skin care products?
- What makes your lesion better and what makes it worse?
- Have you applied any creams, lotions, or gels?
- How often do you bathe and what products do you use?
- Do you have any itching?
- Was the itching immediate or gradual?
- Can you describe the intensity of the itching and the location?
- Is the itching worse at night or at a certain time of year?
- What makes the itching better and what makes it worse?
- Have you applied heat or cold and has that helped?

Assessment: Cardinal Signs and Symptoms

General
- Fever
- Malaise
- Anorexia
- Headache

Head, Eyes, Ears, Nose, Throat (HEENT)
- Red eyes
- Conjunctivitis
- URI

Respiratory
- Asthma
- Allergies
- Cough

Cardiovascular
- Varicosities
- Pedal edema

Gastrointestinal
- Anorexia
- Abdominal pain

Musculoskeletal
- Arthritis
- Joint stiffness

Medical History: General

- Medical conditions, surgeries, and blood transfusions
- Allergies (seasonal as well as others)
- Medication currently used: prescription, birth control pill (BCP), and over-the-counter (OTC) drug
- Herbal preparations and traditional therapies

Medical History: Specific to Complaint

- Childhood asthma or allergies
- Skin cancers or precancers
- Varicella as a child
- Use of sunscreen
- Diabetes
- Psoriasis
- Thyroid or other endocrine disorders
- HIV

Family History

Focus on skin disorders such as atopic dermatitis, psoriasis, seborrheic dermatitis, asthma, hay fever, environmental allergens, persistent rashes, or any inherited skin disorder.

Social History

- Occupation
- Drug and alcohol use
- Outdoor activities, hobbies, or sports
- Military service with focus on type of military occupation

PHYSICAL EXAMINATION

Vital Signs

- Temperature
- Pulse
- Respiration
- Blood pressure (BP)

General Appearance

- Apparent state of health
- Color
- Nutritional status
- State of hydration
- Hygiene
- Older or younger than stated age

Skin, Hair, and Nails

Inspection

- Overall inspection of the skin
- Note skin color
- Inspect the lesion. Is it primary or secondary?
- Identify the size, shape, and elevation of the lesion
- Inspect for the color and arrangement of the lesion
- Note the distribution of the lesion
- Inspect the hair for color, distribution, texture

- Inspect for lesions or infestations in the scalp
- Inspect the nails for color
- Inspect the nails for smoothness and consistency

Palpation
- Palpate the skin for temperature, texture, and moisture
- Assess skin turgor
- Palpate the skin lesion, squeeze, or scrape the lesion
- Palpate the nails for texture, temperature, and tenderness

CASE STUDY
History

Question	Response
Did it start suddenly or come on slowly?	*It was slow*
How long have you had the lesion?	*Probably 9 months*
Do you only have one lesion and where is it located?	*One on my head*
If you have more than one lesion where are they located?	*No*
Can you describe the color, size, and shape of the lesion?	*It is yellow, round, and one inch*
Is the lesion raised?	*I cannot tell*
Is the lesion painful?	*No*
Does the lesion have any drainage? Or, is it crusted or scaling?	*I think scaling, it feels rough*
Has the appearance of the lesion changed since it appeared?	*I think it is worse*
Have you had any fevers, chills, itching, fatigue, or decreased appetite?	*No*
Have you ever had a cancer?	*No*
Have you had any recent injury to your skin or trauma?	*No*
Have you traveled recently?	*No*
Have you been exposed to any chemicals in your home or work?	*No*
Have you been camping, hiking, or working in outdoors?	*I sail almost every day*
Are you taking any medications or drugs?	*Yes, I take BP and diabetes pills*
Have you started any new medications recently?	*No*
Have you had a change in diet or skin care products?	*No*

Question	Response
What makes your lesion better and what makes it worse?	*Nothing*
Have you applied any creams, lotions or gels?	*Jergens lotion after I shower*
How often do you bathe and what products do you use?	*Daily and I use Dove soap*
Do you have any itching?	*A little*
Was the itching immediate or gradual?	*Gradual*
Can you describe the intensity of the itching and the location?	*Not bad*
Is the itching worse at night or at a certain time of year?	*No*
What makes the itching better and what makes it worse?	*Using lotion after I shower*
Have you applied heat or cold and has that helped?	*No*

Physical Examination Findings

- VITAL SIGNS: 98.6°F; heart rate (HR) 82, regular; respiratory rate (RR) 16; BP 128/74
- GENERAL APPEARANCE: well-developed, healthy-appearing tanned male in no acute distress. Appears to be stated age and in good health
- SKIN: tanned, dry skin; scalp—one lesion, 0.5 cm, central scalp, yellow/tan, firm with irregular edge and scaling; proximal to this lesion is another lesion, 0.5 cm, yellow/tan, firm with irregular edge and scaling
- HAIR: male-patterned baldness with white hair
- NAILS: nail and nail fold intact, and adhered to the bed; nails translucent with longitudinal ridging but without grooves or pitting

DIFFERENTIAL DIAGNOSIS

Descriptions	Seborrhea	Rosacea	Cancer	Actinic Keratoses
Color	Red edematous	Dull red	Pale	Pale
Scale	Yes	None	No	No
Smoothness of skin	Yes	Yes	Irregular edges	Scaly irregular surface
Pustules	No	Yes	None	No
Scarring	None	No	None	Yes
Border of lesion	None	No borders	Irregular	Irregular

DIAGNOSTIC EXAMINATION

Examination	Procedure Code	Cost	Results
Scraping	87220	$35 to $50	Identification of nonspecific fungal, nail scrape, or skin using a #15 scalpel blade. Place on slide with a cover slip and apply potassium hydroxide. Direct examination with low light. You may see spores or hyphae. Tzanck smear for herpes virus infection, scrape base of vesicle and place on slide. Apply Giemsa or Wright's stain. Multinucleated giant cells confirm diagnosis. Confirm with viral cultures. Scraping for mites at burrows and place scraping on slide with mineral oil to see the parasite, eggs, or mite feces.
Cultures	87070	$55 to $75	Allows correct identification of microbial organisms of a wound or draining tissue. Collect and grow bacterial, viral, or fungal cultures in appropriate media.
Patch test	95044	$35 to $45	Exposes patient to the most common allergens in patches with 20 of the most common allergens. Apply to skin and removed 2 days later. A positive reaction is eruption at the site of the allergen.
Biopsy	11100	$75 to $95	Shave biopsy is for papular, pedunculated, or exophytic lesions. For inflammatory skin lesions use punch biopsy. Excisional biopsy is used to remove an entire lesion and provides a deeper specimen.

All lesions should be biopsied if there is any doubt.

CLINICAL DECISION MAKING

Case Study Analysis

The advanced practice nurse performs the assessment and physical exam on the patient and finds the following data: a gradual onset of two scalp lesions, 0.5 cm, firm, yellow/tan, and with irregular edges and scaling in an older adult with a history of frequent sun exposure.

> *Diagnosis:* Actinic keratosis

FURTHER READING

Berger, T. G., & Steinhoff, M. (2011). Common dermatoses in the elderly. *Seminars in Cutaneous Medicine and Surgery, 30,* 113–117.

Habif, T. (2005). *Skin disease diagnosis and treatment* (2nd ed.). St. Louis, MO: Mosby.

Henry, G. I., & Caputy, G. (2012, October). *Benign skin lesions overview of benign skin lesions.* Retrieved from http://emedicine.medscape.com/article/1294801-overview

Hess, C. T. (2012). Identifying primary and secondary lesions. *Advances in Skin and Wound Care, 25*(7), 336.

Luggen, A. S. (2003). Wrinkles and beyond: Skin problems in older adults. *Advance Nurse Practitioner,* *11*(60), 55–58.

Rhoads, J., & Petersen, S. W. (2013). *Advanced health assessment and diagnostic reasoning* (2nd ed.). Sudbury, MA: Jones & Bartlett.

Seller, R. H., & Symons, A. B. (2012). *Differential diagnosis of common complaints.* Philadelphia, PA: Elsevier.

Weiss, G. J. (2012). *Diagnosis and treatment of basal cell carcinoma.* Retrieved from http://www .Medscape.org/viewarticle/769560_slide

SKIN RASHES

Case Presentation: *A 45-year-old female presents with a complaint of an itchy red rash on her arms and legs.*

INTRODUCTION TO COMPLAINT

- Skin complaints are very common in primary care settings, it is estimated that 7% of all outpatient visits are for a primary skin complaint.
- Patients with common chronic medical conditions, such as diabetes and obesity, frequently have skin complaints. Yet for primary care clinicians accurately diagnosing skin condition is challenging.
- With skin complaints it is important to be able to accurately identify and describe the characteristics of the skin lesions.
- With skin lesions, the objective findings present in locations are detectable on physical exam.
- With your differential diagnosis of skin lesion, you need to learn how to describe the primary lesion, examine the distribution of the lesions, and be able to describe secondary lesions.

Terms used to describe primary lesions are as follows:

- *Macules* are nonpalpable lesions that vary in pigmentation form the surrounding skin. There are no elevations or depressions of the skin.
- *Papules* are palpable discrete lesions that measure less than 5 mm, presenting as isolated or grouped.
- *Plaques* are larger superficial flat lesions, often forming a confluence of papules.
- *Nodules* are palpable, discrete lesions measuring more than 6 mm, presenting as either an isolated or a grouped lesion. Tumors are considered large nodules.
- *Cysts* are enclosed cavities with a lining that contains a liquid or semisolid material.
- *Pustules* are well-circumscribed papules containing purulent material.
- *Vesicles* are small, less than 5-mm-diameter circumcised papules containing serous material, whereas *Bullae* are larger than 5 mm.
- *Wheals* are irregularly elevated edematous skin areas that are often erythematous.
- *Telangiectasia* is a small superficial dilated blood vessel.
- Secondary lesions are considered evolved lesions or changes. This is due to not having the initial primary disorder not treated.
- *Excoriation* is a linear skin erosion caused by scratching.
- *Lichenification* increases skin thickening with induration secondary to chronic inflammation.

- *Edema* is swelling due to accumulation of water in the tissue.
- *Scale* is superficial dead epidermal cells that are cast off from the skin.
- *Crust* is a scab or dried exudate.
- *Fissure* is a deep skin split that extends into the dermis.
- *Erosion* is a loss of part of the epidermis. These lesions heal without scarring.
- *Atrophy* is decreased skin thickness due to skin thinning.
- *Scar* is an abnormal fibrous tissue that replaces normal tissue after an injury.
- *Hypopigmentation* is a decrease in skin pigment, whereas *depigmentation* is a total loss of skin pigment.

Lesion Location or Distribution

- The distribution of certain lesions is based on the propensity of certain types of lesions or conditions to present in a particular part of the body as well as at a certain age and in certain ethnic groups.
- It is necessary to consider the type of primary lesion, the nature of the secondary lesion, and the distribution of the lesion.

HISTORY OF COMPLAINT
Symptomatology

The following characteristics of each symptom should be elicited and explored using open-ended questions:

- Onset (sudden or gradual)
- Chronology
- Current situation (improving or deteriorating)
- Location
- Radiation
- Quality
- Timing (frequency, duration)
- Severity
- Precipitating and aggravating factors
- Relieving factors
- Associated symptoms
- Effects on daily activities
- Previous diagnosis of similar episodes
- Previous treatments
- Efficacy of previous treatments

Directed Questions to Ask

- How long has the rash/lesion been present?
- How did it look when it first appeared?
- Where did it first appear and where is it now?
- What treatments have been used and what was the response, this time and previously?
- Are any other family members affected or does any family member have a similar history?
- Previous history of similar rash for the patient?
- According to the patient's perspective, what caused the rash?
- Are there any new or different medications, personal care products, occupational or recreational exposures that may have caused the skin lesions/rash?

Additional Questions
- Has been there been any increase in stress in his or her life?
- It is important to obtain a very thorough social history of occupation, hobbies, travel.
- Ask about sun exposure and use of sun protection strategies
- Does the patient have any allergies or potential allergies?
- Have there been any new growths/skin changes?
- Any history of acute blistering sunburns or chronic sun exposure?
- Any history of prior radiation, thermal injury, and cigarette smoking?

Assessment: Cardinal Signs and Symptoms

In addition to the general characteristics outlined above, additional characteristics of specific symptoms should be elicited, as follows:

Skin
- Description of lesion in patient's own words
- Distribution of lesions
- Onset of lesions
- Location of lesions

Other Associated Symptoms
- Fever
- Malaise/fatigue
- Nausea or vomiting

Medical History: General
- Medical conditions and surgeries
- Allergies (seasonal as well as others)
- Medication currently used (prescription, birth control pill [BCP], and over-the-counter [OTC] drug)
- Herbal preparations and traditional therapies

Medical History: Specific to Complaint
- History of chronic illness: diabetes, obesity
- History of autoimmune disorders
- History of skin cancer

PHYSICAL EXAMINATION
Vital Signs
- Temperature
- Pulse
- Respiration
- SpO_2 (oxygen saturation)
- Blood pressure (BP)

General Appearance
- Apparent state of health
- Appearance of comfort or distress
- Color

- Nutritional status
- State of hydration
- Hygiene
- Match between appearance and stated age

Skin

- Type of lesion (see above)
- Shape of individual lesions
- Arrangement of multiple lesions
- Distribution of lesions
- Color
- Consistency

CASE STUDY

History

Question	Response
How long has the rash/lesion been present?	*For about 2 weeks or so*
How did it look when it first appeared?	*Fine slightly raised red dots*
Where did it first appear and where is it now?	*It first appeared on my forearms and now has spread to my abdomen and legs*
What treatments have you used and what was the response, this time and previously?	*I have used aloe vera gel and antibiotic ointment. Aloe vera seems to have helped with the itching.*
Are any other family members affected or have a similar history?	*No*
Have you ever had a rash like this before now?	*I had eczema as a young child; no problem with it as an adult*
What do you think could have caused the rash?	*I think I might have a sun allergy*
Are there any new or different medications, personal care products, occupational or recreational exposures that may have caused the skin lesions/rash?	*I don't take a regular medication, and I work at home as a biller for a physician's office. I was wondering about new spray-on sunscreen.*
Has there been any increase in stress in your life?	*No unusual stress*
Do you have any hobbies or do you travel?	*No new hobbies and I do travel*
Have you had any exposure to the sun and, if so, what form of protection have you used?	*I did go to a local pool with children a lot this summer. I always wore sunscreen and a sunhat.*

Question	Response
Do you have any allergies or potential allergies?	*Some hay fever in the spring; well controlled with antihistamines*
Have there been any new growths/skin changes?	*No*
Any history of acute blistering sunburns, chronic sun exposure?	*No*
Any history of prior radiation, thermal injury and cigarette smoking?	*I smoked in high school and college*

Physical Examination Findings

- VITAL SIGNS: temperature 98.8°F; respiratory rate (RR) 20; heart rate (HR) 88, regular; BP 120/82
- GENERAL APPEARANCE: well-developed, healthy-appearing female in no acute distress
- SKIN: inflammation and mild edema are located on forearms, upper arms, and chest wall, thighs and knees; primary lesions are a macular papular rash with secondary linear excoriations on forearms and legs

DIFFERENTIAL DIAGNOSIS

Differential Diagnosis	Pain	Color	Configuration	Location
Dermatitis	Puritic	Pink to red	Skin eruptions resembling rash	Typically moist areas such as creases of groin or neck or under breasts
Impetigo	Puritic, burning, stinging	Yellow pus-filled vesicles	Leaking pus or fluid, and forms a honey-colored scab, followed by a red mark that heals without leaving a scar.	Nose or mouth
Herpes zoster	Painful	Yellow fluid-filled blisters	Skin rash with blisters	Limited area on one side of the body (left or right), often in a stripe
Eczema	Puritic	Erythematous	Vesicular, weeping, and crusting patches	Face, inside of elbows, under breasts, groin area
Actinic keratosis	None	Dark or light, tan, pink, red, a combination of all these	Thick, scaly, or crusty areas	Sun-exposed areas of body—face, head, neck, arms
Psoriasis	Are usually pruritic	Erythematous	Scaly, patches, papules, and plaques	Elbows, knees, but can affect any area, including the scalp, palms of hands, and soles of feet, and genitals

DIAGNOSTIC EXAMINATION

There are very few diagnostic tests needed to aid in the differential diagnosis of skin conditions. The essential one is the skin biopsy.

Examination	Procedure Code	Cost	Results
Skin biopsy (punch)	11100 11101	$100 $150	• A punch biopsy is considered an excisional biopsy or removes an entire lesion. • This is a procedural code reimbursed at different rates based on the insurance provider. The initial punch is 11100 and each additional is a 11101 code. • A punch biopsy is the primary technique to obtain diagnostic, full-thickness skin specimens. The biopsy is performed using a circular blade. The instrument is rotated down through the dermis and into the subcutaneous fat. The punch biopsy yields a cylindrical core of tissue that must be gently handled to prevent crush debris, which can impact the evaluation of cell pathology. • Large punch biopsy sites can be closed with a single suture and produce a minimal scar. • Punch biopsies are not useful in the evaluation of rashes. They are useful in the differential diagnosis of inflammatory lesions. Punch biopsies are necessary in the evaluation of potentially malignant lesions. If there is a positive finding of malignancy, then additional surgical intervention is necessary and a referral to a dermatologist may be necessary.
Skin biopsy (shave)	11305 (lesion ≤ 0.5 cm) 11306 (lesion, 0.6–1 cm) 11307 (1.1–2 cm) 11308 (lesions > 2 cm)	$150 to $1000 depending on area	• A shave biopsy is an incisional biopsy because it removes only a small part of the lesion. The shave biopsy is used for lesions that are predominantly epidermal without extension into the dermis, such as warts, papillomas, skin tags, superficial basal, or squamous cell carcinomas. A superficial shave removes a think disk of tissue, often by scalpel (usually no. 15 blade) • Excisional biopsies should be performed for any lesions perceived to be melanomas.

CLINICAL DECISION MAKING

Case Study Analysis

The advanced practice nurse performs the assessment and physical examination on the patient and finds a macular papular rash with erythematous base with secondary lesions of excoriations on forearms and legs. The rash has been present for 2 weeks and with discovery of a more detailed history, exposure to spray-on sunscreen appears to be the culprit.

> *Diagnosis:* Irritant contact dermatitis (chronic)

SORE THROAT

Case Presentation: A 35-year-old Asian college student presents to your clinic with a complaint of a sore throat.

INTRODUCTION TO COMPLAINT

Pharyngitis is caused by the following problems:

Viral Infections

- Respiratory syncytial virus
- Influenza A and B
- Epstein–Barr virus (mononuclosis or "kissing disease")
- Adenovirus
- Herpes simplex

Bacterial Infections

- Group A beta strep is the most common bacterial infection of the pharynx
- *Neisseria gonorrhoeae*
- *Mycoplasma pneumonia*
- *Chlamydophila pneumoniae*

Irritants and Injuries

- Low humidity, smoking, air pollution, yelling, or nasal drainage down the back of the throat (postnasal drip)
- Breathing through the mouth when client has allergies or a stuffy nose
- Gastroesophageal reflux disease (GERD)
- An injury to the back of the throat, such as is caused by a cut or puncture from falling with a pointed object in the mouth

HISTORY OF COMPLAINT

Symptomatology

Ask about the following characteristics of each symptom using open-ended questions:

- Onset (gradual or sudden)
- Current situation (improving or deteriorating)
- Location
- Radiation
- Quality

- Timing (frequency, duration)
- Severity
- Precipitating and aggravating factors
- Relieving factors
- Associated symptoms
- Effects on daily activities
- Previous diagnosis of similar episodes
- Previous treatments
- Efficacy of previous treatments

Directed Questions to Ask

- Do you have any fevers?
- Do you have any aches?
- Is it hard to swallow?
- Are you able to drink fluids?
- On a scale of 0 to 10, if 10 is the worse pain you have ever had, what number is this pain?
- Do you have a headache?
- Do you have a rash?
- Do you have fatigue?
- Do you have nasal congestion?
- Do you have a cough?
- Do you have vomiting?
- Have you been exposed to anyone who has sore throat or strep?

Assessment: Cardinal Signs and Symptoms

Ask about the following associated symptoms:

Mouth and Throat
- Hoarseness or recent voice change
- Dental status
- Oral lesions
- Bleeding gums
- Sore throat
- Uvula midline
- Dysphagia

Neck
- Pain
- Swelling
- Enlarged glands

Other Associated Symptoms
- Fever
- Malaise
- Nausea or vomiting

Medical History: General

- Medical conditions and surgeries
- Allergies (seasonal as well as others)
- Medication currently used (prescription, birth control pill [BCP] and over-the-counter [OTC] drug)
- Herbal preparations and traditional therapies

Medical History: Specific to Complaint

- Frequent throat infections
- Sinusitis
- Trauma to the throat area
- History of throat surgery
- Seasonal allergies

PHYSICAL EXAMINATION

Vital Signs

- Temperature
- Pulse
- Respiration
- SpO$_2$ (oxygen saturation)
- Blood pressure (BP)

General Appearance

- Apparent state of health
- Appearance of comfort or distress
- Color
- Nutritional status
- State of hydration
- Hygiene
- Match between appearance and stated age
- Difficulty with gait or balance

Mouth and Throat

Inspection

- Lips: color, lesions, symmetry
- Oral cavity: breath odor, color, lesions of buccal mucosa
- Teeth and gums: redness, swelling, caries, bleeding
- Tongue: color, texture, lesions, tenderness of floor of mouth
- Throat and pharynx: color, exudates, uvula, tonsillar symmetry, and enlargement

Neck Inspection

- Symmetry
- Swelling
- Masses
- Active range of motion
- Thyroid enlargement

Palpation

- Tenderness, enlargement, mobility, contour, and consistency of nodes and masses
- Nodes: pre- and postauricular, occipital, tonsillar, submandibular, submental, anterior and posterior cervical, supraclavicular
- Thyroid: size, consistency, contour, position, tenderness

Associated Systems for Assessment

- A complete assessment should include the respiratory system

CASE STUDY
History

Question	Response
Was the onset sudden or gradual?	*It was sudden*
Have you had any fevers?	*Yes, it was 101 this morning*
Do you have any aches?	*Yes, I am very achy*
Is it hard to swallow?	*Yes, it is so painful*
Are you able to drink fluids?	*Yes, I am drinking some fluids, but it hurts*
If 10 is the worst pain you have ever had, what number is this pain?	*9/10*
Do you have a headache?	*Mild headache here (points to front of head)*
Do you have a rash?	*No*
Do you have fatigue?	*Yes, I am so tired*
Do you have nasal congestion?	*No, I'm not stuffy*
Do you have a cough?	*No, I'm not coughing*
Do you have vomiting?	*No, my stomach is okay*
Have you been exposed to anyone who has sore throat or strep?	*No, not that I know of*

Physical Examination Findings

- VITAL SIGNS: 101°F; respiratory rate (RR) 16; heart rate (HR) 110, regular; BP 100/60
- GENERAL APPEARANCE: Well-developed, healthy appearing female with slightly muffled voice in no acute distress
- EYES: No injection, anicteric, pupils even, round, reactive to light and accommodation (PERRLA), extraocular movements intact
- NOSE: Nares are patent; no edema or exudate of turbinates
- MOUTH: No oral lesions; teeth and gums in good repair.
- PHARYNX: Tonsils are moderately enlarged, red with pockets of white exudate
- NECK: Tonsillar nodes are 1.5 cm, round, mobile, tender bilaterally; no other cervical nodes are palpable; neck is supple; thyroid is not enlarged
- CHEST: Lungs are clear in all fields; heart S1 and S2 has no murmur, gallop, or rub
- ABDOMEN: Soft, nontender without mass or organomegaly
- SKIN: No rashes
- EXTREMITIES: No joint pain or swelling

DIFFERENTIAL DIAGNOSIS

	Viral	Strep	Mono	Postnasal
Onset	Gradual	Abrupt	Either	Gradual
Painful swallowing	+	+	+	+ or −
Fever	Low	High	Either	Low or no
Chills	Rare	+	Either	−
Sweats	Rare	+	Either	−
Nasal congestion	Common	Rare	Rare	Common
Nasal discharge	Common	Rare	Rare	Common
Post nasal drip	Common	Rare	Rare	Common
Cough	Mild	Rare	Rare	Common
Fatigue	Common	Common	Common	Mild
Malaise	Common	Common	Common	Rare
Headache	Mild	Mild	Mild	Mild
Nodes in neck	Boggy	Enlarged tonsillar	Posterior	Boggy
Exposed to strep	Negative	Positive	Negative	Negative

DIAGNOSTIC EXAMINATION

Examination	Procedure Code	Cost	Results
Throat culture (culture usually done when rapid test is negative)	87880 87081	$80 $64	Rapid strep test Normal (negative results): No strep bacteria are present. Abnormal (positive results): Strep bacteria are present. • One problem with the test is that, though it has high specificity of approximately 95% to 98% (http://www.ask .com/wiki/Rapid_strep_test?#cite_note-0), the sensitivity is only 75% to 85% (http://www.ask.com/wiki/Rapid_strep _test?#cite_note-1). • This means that the odds of a false positive are lower than the odds of a false negative and one can be more confident about a positive result than a negative result.

(*continued*)

Examination	Procedure Code	Cost	Results
			• If the rapid test is negative, a follow-up culture (which takes 24 to 48 hours) might be performed. • A negative culture could suggest a viral infection. • Works by detecting the presence of a carbohydrate antigen unique to group A *Streptococcus.* • If the test is performed before sufficient organisms are present in the throat, then the rapid strep test is less likely to detect the organism. • The clinician might still treat the throat infection based on his or her own judgment. Throat culture Normal (negative): No infection (bacteria or fungi) grows in the culture. A negative throat culture may mean the infection is a virus, rather than bacteria or fungus, such as: • Enterovirus • Epstein–Barr virus • Herpes simplex virus • Respiratory syncytial virus Abnormal (positive): Bacteria grow in the culture. Some bacterial throat infections include: • Strep throat • Whooping cough (*Bordetella pertussis*) The most common fungal throat infection is thrush, caused by the fungus *Candida albicans.*
Complete blood count (CBC)	85025	$75	CBC The CBC typically has several parameters: White blood count (WBC) • High WBC can be a sign of infection • WBC is also increased in certain types of leukemia • Low white counts can be a sign of bone marrow diseases or an enlarged spleen. Hemoglobin (Hgb) and hematocrit (Hct) • Hgb is the amount of oxygen-carrying protein contained within the red blood cells (RBCs) • Hct is the percentage of the blood volume by RBCs • Low Hgb or Hct suggests an anemia • High Hgb can occur due to lung disease, living at high altitudes, or excessive bone marrow production of blood cells MCV • Low values suggest iron deficiency; high values suggest deficiencies of either vitamin B_{12} or folate, ineffective production in the bone marrow, or recent blood loss with replacement by newer (and larger) cells from the bone marrow. Platelet count • High values can occur with bleeding, cigarette smoking, or excess production by the bone marrow. • Low values can occur from immune thrombocytopenia, acute blood loss, drug effects (such as heparin), infections with sepsis, entrapment of platelets in an enlarged spleen, or bone marrow failure from myelofibrosis or leukemia.

CLINICAL DECISION MAKING

Case Study Analysis

The advanced practice nurse performs the assessment and physical examination on the patient and finds the following pertinent positives: sudden onset of throat soreness, fever of 101.2°F, chills and malaise, painful swallowing, tonsillar adenopathy, and mastoid adenopathy. Pertinent negatives are absence of runny nose, sinus pain, or cough.

Diagnosis: Strep throat

TINNITIS—RINGING IN THE EARS

Case Presentation: A 77-year-old patient who complains of "ringing in his ears" and states his hearing has gotten progressively worse.

INTRODUCTION TO COMPLAINT

Tinnitus is not a condition itself—it is a symptom of an underlying condition, such as age-related hearing loss, ear injury, or a circulatory system disorder. Causes are:

- Presbycusis: Occurs with aging
- Acoustic trauma: Long exposure to loud noise
- Ear infections: Bacterial or viral infections
- Earwax blockage: Causes hearing loss or irritation of the eardrum, which can lead to tinnitus
- Bony structure changes: Otosclerosis
- Temporomandibular joint (TMJ) disorders: TMJ impairment
- Head injuries or neck injuries: Head or neck trauma, hearing nerves, or brain function linked to hearing
- Acoustic neuroma: This noncancerous (benign) tumor develops on the cranial nerve that runs from the brain to the inner ear and controls balance and hearing; condition generally causes tinnitus in only one ear
- Ototoxicity: A side effect of certain medications or alcohol
- Ménière's disease: Inner ear disorder that may be caused by abnormal inner ear fluid pressure
- Pulsatile tinnitus: Head and neck tumors, atherosclerosis, high blood pressure, turbulent blood flow, and malformation of capillaries

HISTORY OF COMPLAINT

Symptomatology

Ask about the following characteristics of each symptom using open-ended questions:

- Onset (sudden or gradual)
- Chronology
- Current situation (improving or deteriorating)
- Timing (frequency, duration)
- Severity

- Precipitating and aggravating factors
- Relieving factors
- Associated symptoms
- Effects on daily activities
- Previous diagnosis of similar episodes
- Previous treatments
- Efficacy of previous treatments

Directed Questions to Ask

- Was the onset sudden or gradual?
- Is it a continuous problem or does it get better or worse at times?
- Is there any pain associated with the ringing in the ears?
- Have you been feeling fatigued?
- Have you experienced vertigo (a sensation that the room is spinning)?
- Have you experienced any dizziness?
- Have you any difficulty in hearing?
- Have you been feeling confused and falling down; losing your balance?
- Have you been having nausea and vomiting?
- Have you experienced a "full" sensation in the ear?
- Have you experienced any abnormal movements of the eye that can't be controlled?
- Have you had other related symptoms?
- Have any ear drainage?

Assessment: Cardinal Signs and Symptoms

Ear
- Hearing loss
- Ear drainage
- Pain

Neck
- Pain
- Swelling
- Enlarged lymph nodes

Other Associated Symptoms
- Fever
- Malaise
- Nausea or vomiting
- Dizziness

Medical History: General

- Medical conditions and surgeries
- Allergies (seasonal as well as others)
- Medication currently used, including over-the-counter (OTC) medication
- Herbal preparations and traditional therapies

Medical History: Specific to Complaint

- Past ringing in the ears
- Recurrent ear infections

- Recent viral infection or other infection of the respiratory tract
- Recent trauma to the ear

PHYSICAL EXAMINATION
Vital Signs

- Temperature
- Pulse
- Respiration
- SpO_2 (oxygen saturation)
- Blood pressure (BP)

General Appearance

- Apparent state of health
- Appearance of comfort or distress
- Color
- Nutritional status
- State of hydration
- Hygiene
- Match between appearance and stated age
- Difficulty with gait or balance

Ear
- Visual ear exam with otoscope looking for drainage, red edematous tympanic membrane and mobility, ear wax, and structural changes
- Use tuning fork to assess basic hearing: perform Rinne and Weber test

Eyes Inspection
- Vision examination
- Examine pupils of the eyes with pen light
- Extraocular muscles (EOMs)

Nose Inspection
- Inspect nasal passage for drainage, redness, and edema
- Illuminate sinuses

Throat Inspection
- Inspect throat for redness, swollen tonsils, drainage, or exudate

Neck Inspection
- Symmetry
- Swelling
- Masses
- Active range of motion
- Thyroid enlargement

Neuroexamination
- Testing strength of extremities
- Watching patient walk

Cardiac examination
- Check heart sounds, check for murmurs, gallops, and rubs

Respiratory examination
- Check lung sounds for crackles, rales, and wheezing

Palpation
- Palpate sinuses for tenderness; palpate lymph nodes for tenderness, enlargement, mobility, contour, and consistency of nodes and masses
- Nodes: Pre- and postauricular, occipital, tonsillar, submandibular, submental, anterior and posterior cervical, and supraclavicular
- Palpate carotid arteries

Auscultation
- Place stethoscope over the ear, temporal area, or neck to hear any pulsating sound. (If audible, evaluation of vascular system of head and neck to detect vascular tumors.) Auscultate for heart sounds.

CASE STUDY
History

Question	Response
Was the onset sudden or gradual?	*Gradual*
Is it a continuous problem or does it get better or worse at times?	*Continuous*
Is there any pain associated with the ringing in the ears?	*No*
Have you been feeling fatigued?	*No*
Have you experienced vertigo (a sensation that the room is spinning)?	*Yes*
Have you experienced any dizziness?	*Yes*
Have you any difficulty in hearing?	*Yes*
Have you been feeling confused and falling down; losing your balance?	*Yes*
Have you been having nausea and vomiting?	*No*
Have you experienced a "full" sensation in the ear?	*No*
Have you experienced any abnormal movements of the eye that can't be controlled?	*No*
Have you had other related symptoms?	*No*
Having any ear drainage?	*No*

Physical Examination Findings

- VITAL SIGNS: BP 120/80; pulse 72, temperature 98.6°F
- GENERAL APPEARANCE: Healthy appearing, no apparent distress, pleasant
- EARS: Abnormal Weber, abnormal Rinne, cannot hear out of left ear, can hear out of right ear, ringing in left ear only, high-pitched ringing in ears
- EYES: No injection, anicteric, pupils equal, round, and reactive to light and accommodation (PERRLA), and extraocular movements intact
- NOSE: No injection, anicteric, PERRLA, extraocular movements intact
- MOUTH: No oral lesions. Teeth and gums in good repair.
- PHARYNX: Tonsils are moderately enlarged, red with pockets of white exudate.
- NECK: Tonsillar nodes are 1.5 cm, round, mobile, and tender bilaterally. No other cervical nodes palpable. Neck is supple. Thyroid is not enlarged.
- CHEST: Lungs are clear in all fields. Heart S1 and S2 no murmur, gallop, or rub.
- SKIN: Good skin color

DIFFERENTIAL DIAGNOSIS

Differential Diagnosis	Hearing Loss	Ringing in Ears	Dizziness	Ear Drainage	Ear Pain	Fever	Ear Fullness
Presbycusis	+	+ or −	−	−	−	−	−
Acoustic trauma	Common	Common	−	−	−	−	−
Ear infections	+ or −	+ or −	−	Common	Common	Common	+ or −
Earwax blockage	Common	+ or −	−	−	+ or −	−	+ or −
Ear bone changes	+ or −	+ or −	+ or −	−	−	−	−
TMJ disorders	−	+ or −	+ or −	−	+ or −	−	−
Acoustic neuroma	Common	+ or −	+ or −	−	−	−	−
Ototoxicity	Common	Common	Common	−	−	−	−
Ménière's disease	Common	Common	Common	−	−	−	+ or −

DIAGNOSTIC EXAMINATION

Examination	Procedure Code	Cost	Results
Computed tomography (CT) scan of head with contrast	70470	$750 to $950	CT yields cross-sectional images of a part of the head through computerized axial tomography

(continued)

Examination	Procedure Code	Cost	Results
Complete blood count (CBC)	85025	$75	**CBC** • The CBC typically has several parameters that are created from an automated cell counter. The most relevant are: **White blood count (WBC)** • The number of white cells • High WBC can be a sign of infection • WBC is also increased in certain types of leukemia • Low WBC can be a sign of bone marrow diseases or an enlarged spleen • Low WBC is also found in HIV infection in some cases. (*Editor's note:* The vast majority of low WBC in our population is not HIV related.) **Hemoglobin (Hgb) and hematocrit (Hct)** • Hgb is the amount of oxygen-carrying protein contained within the red blood cells (RBCs). • Hct is the percentage of the blood volume occupied by RBCs. **MCV** • Identify cause of an anemia: Low values suggest iron deficiency; high values suggest deficiencies of either vitamin B_{12} or folate, ineffective production in the bone marrow, or recent blood loss. **Platelet count** • High values can occur with bleeding, cigarette smoking. Low values can occur from premature destruction or excess production by the bone marrow. • States such as immune thrombocytopenia, acute blood loss, drug effects (such as heparin), infections with sepsis, entrapment of platelets in an enlarged spleen, or bone marrow failure from diseases such as myelofibrosis or leukemia.
Basic metabolic panel (BMP)	80047	$160	The BMP includes the following tests: • Glucose: Abnormal levels can indicate diabetes or hypoglycemia. Glucose: 64 to 128 mg/dL • Calcium: Essential for the proper functioning of muscles, nerves, and the heart and is required in blood clotting and in the formation of bones. Elevated or decreased calcium levels may indicate a hormone imbalance or problems with the kidneys, bones, or pancreas. Serum calcium: 8.5 to 10.2 mg/dL • Sodium: Vital nerve and muscle function; serum sodium: 136 to 144 mEq/L • Potassium: Cell metabolism and muscle function; serum potassium: 3.7 to 5.2 mEq/L • CO_2 (carbon dioxide, bicarbonate): Maintains the body's acid–base balance (pH). CO_2 (carbon dioxide): 20 to 29 mmol/L

Examination	Procedure Code	Cost	Results
Basic metabolic panel (BMP) (*continued*)			• Chloride: Regulates the amount of fluid in the body and maintains the acid–base balance. Serum chloride: 101 to 111 mmol/L • BUN (blood urea nitrogen): Conditions that affect the kidney have the potential to affect the amount of urea in the blood. BUN: 7 to 20 mg/dL • Creatinine: Waste product produced in the muscles; filtered out of the blood by the kidneys so blood levels are a good indication of how well the kidneys are working. Creatinine: 0.8 to 1.4 mg/dL
EKG	93000	$800	An EKG is a test that records the electrical activity of the heart. It is used to measure: • Heart rate • The effects of drugs or devices used to control the heart (such as a pacemaker) • The size and position of heart • Abnormal heart rhythms • Damage or changes to the heart muscle • Changes in the amount of sodium or potassium in the blood • Congenital heart defect • Enlargement of the heart • Fluid or swelling around the heart • Myocarditis • Past or current myocardial infarction (MI)

CLINICAL DECISION MAKING

Case Study Analysis

Patient has had a recent fall that resulted in a fractured clavicle and progressive hearing loss. Patient has experienced dizziness and loss of balance. Physical examination reveals an abnormal Rinne and Weber test and abnormal EKG with frequent premature atrial contractions and premature ventrical contractions noted.

> *Diagnosis:* Alteration in hearing related to hearing loss and tinnitus confirmed by physical examination and assessment with positive Rinne and Weber test. Diagnostic examinations will determine further issues. The patient will need to be referred to the ear/nose/throat physician for his hearing loss associated with the above symptoms, which may be due to a neurosensory hearing loss.

FURTHER READING

Rhoads, J., & Petersen, S. (2013). *Advanced health assessment and diagnostic reasoning* (2nd ed.). Sudbury, MA: Jones & Bartlett.

VAGINAL DISCHARGE

Case Presentation: *A 33-year-old married female presents to the clinic with a vaginal discharge associated with a strong odor for the past 3 days.*

INTRODUCTION TO COMPLAINT

A vaginal discharge may be caused by a bacterial infection, a retained tampon, or vaginal dryness from atrophic vaginitis.

Infectious Process

Bacterial Vaginitis
- Alkaline vaginal pH due to menstrual blood, semen, or decrease in lactobacilli
- Poor perineal hygiene, especially in patients who are incontinent or have limited mobility
- Chemicals in the bubble bath or soap
- Introduction of foreign objects
- Low estrogen can be a predisposing factor for vaginitis
- Use of antibiotics
- Pregnancy
- Diabetes mellitus

Candidal Vaginitis
- An overgrowth of bacteria of the normal flora
- Causes alteration in vaginal pH
- Discharge looks like cottage cheese and adheres to the vaginal wall
- Sometimes worsens after intercourse and before menses
- Recent antibiotic use or history of diabetes
- Identified by a vaginal pH < 4.5 with identifications of yeast or hyphae on a wet mount or potassium hydroxide (KOH) preparation

Trichomonal Vaginitis
- Caused by the protozoan *Trichomonas vaginalis*
- A sexually transmitted disease that presents with discharge that is diffuse, malodorous, and yellow–green with irritation

Atrophic Vaginitis
- Most common cause of vaginitis
- Discharge associated with atrophic vaginitis
- May be initially misdiagnosed as a yeast infection
- Discharge does not have a foul odor
- The microscopic examination is negative for findings indicative of yeast or common bacterial infections

Cervicitis
- Resembles vaginitis
- Abdominal pain, cervical motion tenderness, or cervical inflammation suggests pelvic inflammatory disease (PID)

Noninfectious Process

- Hypersensitivity or irritant reactions to hygiene sprays or perfumes, menstrual pads, laundry soaps, bleaches, fabric softeners, fabric dyes, synthetic fibers, bathwater additives, toilet tissue, or, occasionally, spermicides, vaginal lubricants or creams, latex condoms, vaginal contraceptive rings, or diaphragms
- A retained tampon is another common cause of vaginal odor and discharge

HISTORY OF COMPLAINT

Symptomatology

Ask about the following characteristics of each symptom using open-ended questions:

- Onset, gradual or abrupt
- Location of the discharge, vaginal or rectal
- Timing and frequency
- Aggravating or triggering factors
- Alleviating factors
- Pain associated with the discharge
- Effects on daily life

Directed Questions to Ask

- When did the change or abnormal vaginal discharge begin?
- Do you have the same amount and type of vaginal discharge throughout the month?
- What does the discharge look like (color and consistency)?
- Is there an odor?
- Do you have pain, itching, or burning?
- Does your sexual partner have a discharge as well?
- Do you have multiple sexual partners or sexual partners that you do not know very well?
- What type of birth control do you use?
- Do you use condoms?
- Is there anything that relieves the discharge?
- Have you tried over-the-counter creams? Have they helped?
- Do you douche?
- Do you have any other symptoms like abdominal pain, vaginal itching, fever, vaginal bleeding, rash, genital warts or lesions, or changes in urination like difficulty, pain, or blood?
- Have you recently changed the detergents or soaps that you use?
- Do you frequently wear very tight clothing?

Assessment: Cardinal Signs and Symptoms

- Foul-smelling, white, cheesy discharge
- Painful intercourse

Medical History: General

- Current medical problems
- Past medical problems

- Past surgeries
- Current medications
- Medication allergies
- Family history
- Social history

Medical History: Specific to Complaint

- Menstrual history
- History of numerous sex partners
- Unprotected sex
- History of STDs in past 2 years

PHYSICAL EXAMINATION

Inspection and Palpation of the External Genitalia

- The external genitalia are examined, some mild erythema and irritation noted on the labia
- There is no swelling or blood noted
- The inguinal nodes are palpated and no tenderness noted
- Some discharge is noted on the vagina that is thick, milky, and gray in color, with a fishy odor

Speculum Assessment of the Internal Genitalia and Inspection of the Vaginal Wall

- The vaginal is wall noted to have some discharge
- No pain on insertion of the speculum, the cervix is normal in color
- Vaginal pH is measured and samples and secretions are taken for assessment. A high pH above 4.5 is associated with bacterial vaginosis. A pH below 4.5 is normal.

Bimanual Examination

No cervical motion tenderness and adnexal or uterine tenderness. The uterus is palpable.

CASE STUDY

History

Question	Response
Describe the discharge	*It was gray to greenish*
When was the onset and duration?	*About 3 days ago*
Is there an odor?	*Yes*
Are the symptoms associated with your period?	*No*
Are you experiencing pain? If yes, when?	*No, no pain, perhaps a little irritation in the vagina with sex*
Do you have itching, rash?	*No*

Physical Examination Findings

- VITAL SIGNS: BP 120/80, temperature 98.6°F, respiratory rate (RR) 18, heart rate (HR) 68
- GENERAL APPEARANCE: Healthy young female
- Skin is warm, dry; no lesions, or acne
- Good hygiene
- Weight 123 lbs; height 5'2"
- Has sexual intercourse with husband at least once a week, not using any lubricant
- Last Pap smear was a year ago and was normal
- Vaginal discharge is milky, gray in color with a "terrible," fishy odor; denies any blood, pain, or burning when urinating; no noticeable redness, irritation, lesion, or wound in the vaginal area
- Current medications include calcium pills

DIFFERENTIAL DIAGNOSIS

	Bacterial Vaginitis	Candida	Trichomoniasis
Discharge	Yes	Yes	Yes
Color/characteristics	White, gray, or yellow	White, cheesy	Frothy yellow or greenish
Odor	Fishy	No	Foul
Pain	No	On intercourse, around vulva	On urination
Other symptoms	Itching, burning, redness, swelling of vulva/vagina	Itching, burning, vulvar swelling	Itching, burning

DIAGNOSTIC EXAMINATION

Examination	Procedure Code	Cost	Results
KOH	87210	$10.53	• Two-slide preparation: (a) 10% KOH, (b) normal saline (NS) • 10% KOH slide: will be positive for fishy odor 76% of the time in the presence of bacterial vaginitis (BV; whiff test) • Examine under microscope for branching and budding hyphae—characteristic of yeast (*Candida*) infection • Clue cells (epithelial cells imbedded with bacteria) are characteristic of BV • NS slide: Examine under microscope for motile trichomonads that signal the presence of *Trichomonas*
pH testing	83986	$7.90	• Using litmus paper: normal vaginal secretions have pH < 4.5 • A higher pH is consistent with BV, trichomoniasis, or atrophic vaginitis • pH of 4.0 to 4.7 consistent with *Candida* • pH of 6.5 to 7.0 may indicate atrophic vaginitis (if few white blood cells [WBCs] and negative for pathogens)

(*continued*)

Examination	Procedure Code	Cost	Results
Wet mount	87070	$23.26	• If pH < 4.5, wet mount reveals up to three to five WBCs/high power field and the presence of epithelial cells and lactobacilli (may be physiological discharge) • WBCs high in the presence of foreign body

CLINICAL DECISION MAKING

Case Study Analysis

The following pertinent positives were found: patient reports milky gray fishy-smelling discharge ongoing for 3 days. Menses are regular. pH is elevated and there is a positive whiff test with clue cells present on microscopy. Pertinent negatives are no pain with sexual intercourse, no itching, burning, or swelling of vagina. No new sexual partner. No budding yeast or mycelia present on microscopic examination.

> **Diagnosis:** *Bacterial vaginosis*

FURTHER READING

Barad, D. H. (2012). *Vaginal itching and discharge.* Retrieved from http://www.merckmanuals.com/professional/gynecology_and_obstetrics/symptoms_of_gynecologic_disorders/vaginal_itching_and_discharge.html

Bickley, L. S. (2009). Female genitalia. In L. S. Bickley (Eds.), *Bates' guide to physical examination and history taking* (pp. 195–280). Philadelphia, PA: Lippincott.

CPT codes and fees. Pathology and laboratory. (2013). Retrieved from http://www.ic.nc.gov/ncic/pages/80000.htm

Dains, J. E., Baumann, L. C., & Scheibel, P. (2007). *Advanced health assessment and clinical diagnosis in primary care* (3rd ed.). St. Louis, MO: Elsevier Science.

VAGINAL LESIONS

Case Presentation: A 19-year-old female reports to you that she has "sores" on and in her vagina. She tries to practice safe sex but has a steady boyfriend and figures she doesn't need to be so careful since she is on the birth control pill (BCP).

INTRODUCTION TO COMPLAINT

Sores in the perineal area can be painless or painful. Several sexually transmitted infections (STIs) are the most common cause of these sores.

Viral Infections

- Caused by a viral infection, such as herpes simplex virus (HSV-I, HSV-II) or human papillomavirus
- Transmitted through intimate contact with a person who is shedding the virus
- Herpes simplex viral infection can be triggered by stress
- Other viral infections, such as molluscum contagiosum or chlamydia

Bacterial Infections

- A bacterial infection, such as syphilis
- Transmitted through unprotected sexual intercourse with an infected person
- Other infections, such as chancroid or granuloma inguinale

Irritants and Injuries

- Sores in the perineal area also can be caused by some kind of trauma.
- These are usually transmitted from person to person through unprotected sex.
- A person can be infected and not know it; the sores may be triggered by some kind of event, such as hormonal stimuli, stress, or menstruation.

HISTORY OF COMPLAINT

Symptomatology

Ask about the following characteristics of each symptom using open-ended questions:

- Chronology
- Current situation (improving or deteriorating)
- Location
- Radiation

- Quality
- Timing (frequency, duration)
- Severity
- Precipitating and aggravating factors
- Relieving factors
- Associated symptoms
- Effects on daily activities
- Previous diagnosis of similar episodes
- Previous treatments
- Efficacy of previous treatments

Directed Questions to Ask

- When did you first notice the sores?
- Was the onset sudden or gradual?
- Are the sores itchy?
- Have you had any swelling, burning, or redness?
- Are the sores painful?
- If 10 is the worse pain you have ever had, what number is the pain?
- Do you have any drainage from the sores?
- Do you have any rashes on your palms or soles of your feet?
- Have you had any fevers?
- Have you noticed these sores anywhere else?
- Have you noticed a foul smelling discharge?
- Do you use condoms during sexual intercourse?
- Have you ever been diagnosed with an STI? If so, what was it?
- Has your boyfriend ever been diagnosed with an STI? If so, what was it?
- Are both you and your boyfriend committed to a monogamous relationship?
- When was your last Pap smear? Have you ever had any abnormal results?

Assessment: Cardinal Signs and Symptoms

Genital/Urinary

- Pain or difficulty when urinating
- Urinary tract infection
- Blood in urine
- Length and time of menstrual cycle
- Vaginal bleeding; how long and how much
- Foul or yellow/green vaginal discharge
- Vaginal lesions
- Vaginal infections

Medical History: General

- Medical conditions and surgeries
- History of allergies
- Medications currently prescribed and over the counter (OTC)
- Herbal preparations and traditional therapies

Medical History: Specific to Complaint

- History of vaginal infections?
- Trauma to vaginal area?
- History of surgery in vaginal area?

- History of urinary tract infections?
- History of STIs?
- Last Pap smear? What were the results?
- Have you ever been pregnant? If so, how many children? Any living children?
- Have you ever had an abortion?

PHYSICAL EXAMINATION
Vital Signs

- Temperature
- Pulse
- Respiration
- Blood pressure (BP)

General Appearance

- Apparent state of health
- Appearance of comfort or distress
- Color
- Nutritional status
- State of hydration
- Hygiene

Genital/Urinary Inspection
- Skin: Note the color, texture
- Mons pubis, labia majora and minora, urethral meatus, clitoris, vaginal introitus, and perineum: Note any inflammation, excoriation, ulceration, discharge, swelling, or nodules
- Vagina, vaginal walls: Note the color, and any inflammation, ulceration, discharge, swelling, or nodules
- Cervix: Note the color, position, characteristics of the surface, and any ulcerations, nodules, masses, bleeding, or discharge. Palpate the cervix to check position, shape, consistency, regularity, mobility, and tenderness
- Uterus, ovaries: Palpate the size, shape, consistency, and mobility. Note any tenderness or masses
- Pelvic muscles: Check for strength, tenderness during contraction, appropriate relaxation after contraction and endurance

Palpation
- Any nodules or lumps (inguinal nodes)? Note the size, consistency, position, and tenderness

CASE STUDY
History

Question	Response
When did you first notice the sores?	*3 months ago*
Was the onset sudden or gradual?	*Gradual*
Are the sores itchy?	*No*

Question	Response
Have you had any swelling, burning, or redness?	*Swelling and burning during urination*
Are the sores painful?	*Yes, very, during intercourse and urination*
If 10 is the worse pain you have ever had, what number is the pain?	*5.5*
Do you have any drainage from the sores?	*Yes, there is yellowish discharge from the sores that comes and goes*
Do you have any rashes on your palms or soles of your feet?	*No*
Have you had any fevers?	*Yes, I have a fever now and had a fever of 100°F yesterday*
Have you noticed these sores anywhere else?	*Yes, I have bumps on the inner creases of my thighs and pelvic area*
Have you noticed a foul smelling discharge?	*No*
Do you use condoms during sexual intercourse?	*No*
Have you even been diagnosed with an STI?	*No*
Has your boyfriend ever been diagnosed with an STI? If so, what was it?	*Not that I know of*
Are both you and your boyfriend committed to a monogamous relationship?	*Yes, we have been committed for the past year*
When was your last Pap smear?	*My first and only Pap smear was 3 years ago when I was 16 years old. I received birth control from a free clinic that does not require pelvic examinations for prescription refills*
Have you ever had any abnormal results?	*No*
What types of food do you usually eat?	*I eat a lot of junk food*
How many glasses of water do you drink a day?	*I don't drink water, but drink a lot of Diet Coke*

Physical Examination Findings

- VITAL SIGNS: temperature: 100.2°F; pulse 72; respirations 18; BP 130/88; weight 156 lbs, 25 lbs overweight; height 5'3"
- GENERAL APPEARANCE: patient appears to have good hygiene; minimal makeup, pierced ears, no tattoos; well nourished (slightly overweight); no obvious distress noted

- CARDIAC: within normal limits, heart rate regular in rhythm
- RESPIRATORY: within normal limits, appropriate lung sounds auscultated, clear and equal bilaterally
- GASTROINTESTINAL: tender during palpation; the left lower quadrant was very tender during palpation; patient denies nausea or vomiting
- INTEGUMENTARY: hot and dry; skin turgor has fast recoil, no tenting noted
- MUSCULOSKELETAL: poor muscle tone; full range of motion of all extremities; no muscle deformities; no history of broken bones prior to fractured femur
- VAGINAL: labia major and minor: numerous ulcerations, too many to count; some ulcerations enter the vaginal introitus; no ulcerations in the vagina mucosa; cervix is clear, some greenish discharge; bimanual exam reveals tenderness in left lower quadrant; able to palpate the left ovary; unable to palpate the right ovary; no tenderness; uterus is normal in size, slight tenderness with cervical mobility
  - No odor; whiff test is negative
  - No history of pregnancy or abortion
- INGUINAL LYMPH NODES: tenderness bilaterally, numerous, 1 cm in size
  - Four palpated on right side and three palpated on left side

DIFFERENTIAL DIAGNOSIS

Differential Diagnoses	Syphilis	Genital Warts	Herpes	Pelvic Inflammatory Disease	Molluscum Contagiosum
Painful	No	No	Yes	Yes	No
Lesions	Yes	Yes	Yes	No	Yes
Itchiness	No	Yes	Yes	No	Yes
Vaginal discharge	No	Yes	Yes	Yes	No
Sexually transmitted	Yes	Yes	Yes	Yes	Yes
Rashes	Yes	No	No	No	No

DIAGNOSTIC EXAMINATIONS

Examination	Procedure Code	Cost	Results
Serology for syphilis	RPR VDRL EIA 2007443	$49 to $79	Detects antibodies for the bacteria that cause syphilis Results in 1 to 4 days
Viral culture; Tzanck smear	88160	$80 to $100?	Rapid diagnostic test used to identify cells from suspected herpes lesions Results available in 1 to 5 days

(continued)

Examination	Procedure Code	Cost	Results
PAP smear ThinPrep	2000137	$5 to $33	A microscopic examination of the cells scraped from the cervical opening Results in 1 to 14 days
Beta human chorionic gonadotropin (hCG), urine qualitative	81025	Tests for pregnancy	Results available in 24 hours

CLINICAL DECISION MAKING

Case Study Analysis

Patient has a fever of 100°F, ulcerated sores with a yellowish discharge causing pain of 5 out of 10, lower left abdominal pain, cervix with greenish discharge, tenderness with cervical mobility, burning on urination, and tenderness of inguinal nodes (~1 cm in size)—four on right side and three on left side.

> **Diagnosis:** *Genital herpes*

FURTHER READING

Bickley, L. S. (2009). *Bates' guide to physical examination and history taking* (10th ed.). Philadelphia, PA: Lippincott.

Dains, J. E., Baumann, L. C., & Scheibel, P. (2007). *Advanced health assessment and clinical diagnosis in primary care* (3rd ed.). St. Louis, MO: Elsevier Science.

McCance, K., Huether, S., Brashers, V., & Rote, N. (2010). *Pathophysiology: The biologic basis for disease in adults and children* (6th ed.). Maryland Heights, MO: Mosby Elsevier.

VOMITING

Case Presentation: *A 16-year-old female comes to the clinic with her mother because of frequent vomiting for the past 4 months.*

INTRODUCTION TO COMPLAINT

Vomiting is a symptom and is associated with the following disorders:

- *Peptic ulcer disease*: This is a constant burning pain that may be accompanied by nausea, vomiting.
- *Viral gastroenteritis*: This can occur at any age and usually involves a diffuse, cramping pain along with nausea, vomiting, diarrhea, and low-grade fever. It usually resolves on its own.
- *Bowel obstruction*: Sudden onset of crampy pain usually in umbilical area of epigastrium. Vomiting occurs early with small intestinal obstruction and late with large bowel obstruction.
- *Ileus*: Abdominal distention, vomiting, obstipation, and cramping due to a decreased peristalsis.
- *Acute pancreatitis*: Usually presents with a history of cholelithiasis or alcohol abuse. Pain is steady and boring and is unrelieved by change in position, located in the left upper quadrant and radiates to back; nausea, vomiting, and diaphoresis.
- *Acute cholelithiasis or cholecystitis*: Appears in adults more than children, females more than males, colicky pain progressing to constant pain; located in right upper quadrant that may radiate to right scapular area; pain of cholelithiasis is constant, progressively rising to plateau and falling gradually; nausea, vomiting, history of dark urine and/or light stools.
- *Renal calculi*: Sudden-onset, excruciating colicky pain that may progress to constant pain. Pain in lower abdomen and flank and radiates to groin; nausea, vomiting, abdominal distention, chills and fever, increased frequency of urination.
- *Pyelonephritis*: Fever, chills, back pain, nausea and vomiting, toxic appearance. Sometimes frequency and dysuria are associated with pyelonephritis.
- *Salmonella food poisoning*: Acute onset 12 to 24 hours after exposure; lasts 2 to 5 days; moderate to large amounts of nonbloody diarrhea, abdominal cramping, and vomiting.
- *Enteromoeba histolytica*: Acute onset 8 to 18 hours after ingestion of contaminated food or water, large amounts of bloody diarrhea, abdominal cramping, and vomiting.
- *Diabetic enteropathy*: Nocturnal diarrhea, postprandial vomiting, fatty stools from malabsorption caused by poorly controlled diabetes.
- *Diabetic ketoacidosis*: Excessive thirst, frequent urination, nausea and vomiting, abdominal pain, weakness or fatigue, shortness of breath, fruity scented breath, and confusion.
- *Pregnancy*: Delayed or irregular menses with sexual activity and no contraception.

- *Brain tumor*: Headaches; nausea and vomiting; changes in speech, vision, or hearing; problems balancing or walking; changes in mood or personality; problems with memory; muscle jerking or twitching; numbness, or tingling in the arms or legs.
- *Appendicitis*: Peaks at age 10 to 20 years. Sudden onset of colicky pain that progresses to a constant pain. The pain may begin in epigastrium or periumbilicus and later localizes to the right lower quadrant (RLQ). Pain worsens with movement or coughing. Vomiting after the onset of pain sometimes occurs. The patient will demonstrate involuntary guarding. Classically, pain occurs in the RLQ. Tests for peritoneal irritation will be positive. Rebound tenderness will be present. Variation in presentation is common, especially in infants, children, and the elderly.

HISTORY OF COMPLAINT
Symptomatology

Ask about the following characteristics of each symptom using open-ended questions:

- Is onset gradual or abrupt?
- Duration, timing, and frequency
- Presence of abdominal pain and location
- Can you describe the abdominal pain?
- Characteristics of emesis
- What triggers or aggravates the desire to vomit?
- What alleviates vomiting? Have you tried anything?
- How has this affected your lifestyle?

Directed Questions to Ask

- Are you sexually active?
- When was your last period?
- Have you had any pain with intercourse?
- Have you had a vaginal discharge or abnormal bleeding?
- Do you vomit at certain times of the day, such as the morning?
- Do you wake up at night to vomit?
- Do you vomit more when you eat certain foods, like fatty or fried foods?
- Do you have any burning in the stomach or chest?
- Is there pain anywhere in your abdominal area?
- Do you have any pain in the back?
- Do you have pain with urination?
- Is there any stress in your life right now?

Assessment: Cardinal Signs and Symptoms

Ask about the following associated symptoms.

Genitourinary
- Description of any pain
- Last menstrual period
- Regularity of periods

Gastrointestinal
- Bowel function
- Appetite
- Weight loss

Other Associated Symptoms
- Activities of daily living

Medical History: General

- Medical history
- Surgical history
- Family history
- Social history, including smoking, alcohol, use of drugs, occupation, hobbies, marital status
- Allergies to medications
- Medication currently used

Medical History: Specific to Complaint

- History of new medications such as aspirin, ibuprofen, or naprosyn
- Family history of gastrointestinal diseases
- Exposure to anyone with similar symptoms

PHYSICAL EXAMINATION

Vital Signs

Take temperature/pulse/respiration and blood pressure. Take blood pressure supine, sitting, and standing.

General Appearance

- EYES: observe for icteric sclera
- MOUTH: observe for dry mucus membranes
- NECK: inspect for abnormal lymph nodes
- CHEST: listen to heart for the rate and rhythm, and the presence of abnormal sounds
- LUNGS: listen for crackles that may indicate a lower lobe pneumonia
- ABDOMEN: inspect for previous scars, abdominal distention, or hernias; listen to the bowel tones in all quadrants and note if active, hyperactive, or hypoactive; palpate the last painful area first with light and then deep palpation; assess for enlargement of the liver, spleen, or kidneys as well as any unusual masses
- RECTAL EXAMINATION: check for frank or occult blood in the stool
- EXTREMITIES: note whether edema is present

CASE STUDY

History

Question	Response
When did you start vomiting?	*A few months ago*
Was it sudden?	*Yes, I woke up one morning with it*
Is there a color?	*It is clear, or it is what I just ate*
Is there any blood in it?	*No, never*
Do you have any fevers?	*No, I feel okay otherwise*

Question	*Response*
Do you have any pain in your belly area?	*No, nothing hurts*
Does anything make it worse?	*Yes, the smell of bacon or fried meats*
Does anything make it better?	*Yes, resting or sipping cola*
Do you have any diarrhea or constipation?	*No, I go okay*
Is it worse with fried foods?	*I don't like fried foods*
Is it worse with milk?	*No, milk is fine*
Do you keep any food or fluids down?	*Yes, small amounts, I nibble*
Do you have a burning feeling anywhere?	*No*
Do you have menstrual periods?	*Yes, since I was 14*
Are they regular?	*No, they have never been regular*
Have you ever had sex with anyone?	*No, that would be against our religion*
Do you have any vaginal discharge?	*No*
Do you have any unusual bleeding?	*No*
Do you have any back pain?	*No*
Do you have any pain with urination?	*No*
Do you drink alcohol?	*No*
Do you smoke?	*No*
Do you use any drugs?	*No*
Do you take any medications?	*No*
Have you had any surgery on your belly?	*No*
Mom, is there any family history of vomiting?	*No, she's the only one like this*

Physical Examination Findings

- VITAL SIGNS: temperature 97°, heart rate (HR) 88, respiratory rate (RR) 16, blood pressure (BP) 110/70
- GENERAL APPEARANCE: anxious shy female; mom is asked to leave the room during the examination
- EYES: anicteric
- MOUTH: mucus membrane is moist
- NECK: no lymphadenopathy
- CHEST: heart has normal S1 and S2, no murmur
- LUNGS: clear and resonant without labored breathing
- ABDOMEN: soft, flat with normal bowel tones; nontender, no organomegaly or masses
- PELVIC: external, shows no abnormal lesions; bulbo-urethral and skenes glands negative
- VAGINAL: smooth walls with normal rugae; no vaginal discharge
- CERVIX: nulliparous, no cervical motion tenderness
- OVARIES: nonpalpable
- UTERUS: enlarged, smooth, nontender, size 12 weeks
- EXTREMITIES: no edema

DIFFERENTIAL DIAGNOSIS

Differential Diagnosis	Infection	Food Poisoning	Obstruction	Metabolic Disorder	Appendicitis	Pregnancy	Cholecystitis/ Pancreatitis
Onset: gradual/rapid	Rapid	Rapid	Gradual	Gradual	Gradual	Gradual	Rapid
Nausea/ vomiting	Nausea and vomiting	Nausea and vomiting	Nausea and possible vomiting depending on location of obstruction	Nausea and vomiting	Nausea and vomiting	Nausea, vomiting intermittent, typically in the morning	Nausea, vomiting intermittent
Malaise	Yes	Yes	Yes	Yes	Yes	None	None
Fever	Possible	Possible	Possible	None	Typically low grade	None	Possible
Diarrhea	Possible	Possible	Possible	None	None	None	None
Bowel sounds, + or –	Hyperactive	Hyperactive	Areas of hyper activity and hypoactivity	Hyperactive	Hyperactive	Normal	Normal
Abdominal pain, + or –	All quadrants	All quadrants	Possible around obstruction	Upper abd. pain	Midline initially, then moves to RLQ	None	Upper right quadrant or epigastric
Liver enlarged	Possible	Possible	Possible	Possible	None	None	Possible
Abnormal laboratory parameters	Elevated white blood cell (WBC)	Elevated WBC	Elevated WBC	Elevated WBC	Elevated WBC	None	Elevated WBC, elevated lipase

DIAGNOSTIC EXAMINATION

Examination	Procedure Code	Cost	Results
Complete blood count (CBC)	85025	$10.69	CBC: • White blood count (WBC): White blood cells protect the body against infection. When there is an infection present, the WBC rises very quickly. The WBC includes a differential white count. • WBC differential: ▪ Neutrophils: The most abundant of the white blood cells. They respond more rapidly to areas of tissue injury and are active during an acute infection. ▪ Eosinophils: Are active during allergic or parasitic illnesses ▪ Basophils: Will increase during the healing process ▪ Monocytes: The second defense mechanism against bacterial and inflammatory illnesses; monocytes are slower to respond than neutrophils but are bigger and can ingest larger molecules. ▪ Lymphocytes: Become increased after chronic bacterial and viral infections • Red blood cells (RBCs): These cells carry O_2 from the lungs to the body. • Hematocrit: This is the measure of the amount of space the RBCs take up in the blood. • Hemoglobin: This is the molecule that fills up the RBCs. • Mea corpuscular volume (MCV): Shows the size of the RBCs • Mean cell hemoglobin (MCH): Shows the amount of hemoglobin contained in the average RBC • Mean corpuscular hemoglobin concentration (MCHC): Measures the concentration of the hemoglobin in an average RBC • Platelets: The platelets play an important role in blood clotting.
Lipase	83690	$9.47	• Elevated level: Indicates possible acute pancreatitis, chronic pancreatitis, cancer of the pancreas, obstruction of the pancreatic duct, perforated ulcer, and acute renal failure.
Complete metabolic panel (CMP)	80053	$14.53	• Glucose level: Is used to determine a possible diagnosis of a prediabetic state or diabetes mellitus. • Creatinine clearance: Decreased levels could be an indicator of renal impairment. • Alkaline phosphatase, alanine aminotransferase, aspartate aminotransferase: These are all diagnostic tests that indicate how the liver is functioning.
Urine pregnancy	84703	$10.33	• Determines whether patient is pregnant

Examination	Procedure Code	Cost	Results
Urinalysis	81003	$3.09	• Color: ■ Red or red–brown: Indication of possible blood in urine, foods such as beets, or medication ■ Orange: Restricted fluid intake, concentrated urine, medications, and foods such as carrots ■ Blue or green: *Pseudomonas* toxemia, medications, or yeast concentrate ■ Black or dark brown: Lysol poisoning, melanin, bilirubin, medications • Appearance: Hazy or cloudy appearance can indicate bacteria, white blood cell (WBC), phosphates. Milky appearance indicates fat or pyuria. • Odor: Ammonia—urea breakdown by bacteria; foul—due to bacteria; sweet or fruity—diabetic ketoacidosis • Foam: Liver cirrhosis, bilirubin, or bile • pH: < 4.5 = acidosis or diet high in meat; > 8 = bacteriuria, urinary tract infection (UTI) • Specific gravity: < 1.005 = diabetes insipidus, excess fluid intake, overhydration, renal disease, severe potassium deficit; > 1.026 = decreased fluid intake, fever, diabetes mellitus, vomiting, diarrhea, dehydration • Protein: > 8 = proteinuria, exercise, severe stress, fever, acute infectious disease, renal disease, lupus, cardiac disease, septicemia • Glucose: > 15 = diabetes mellitus, central nervous system (CNS) disorders, stroke, Cushing's syndrome, glucose infusions, severe stress, infections • Ketones: +1 to +3 = ketoacidosis, starvation, diet high in proteins • Red blood cells (RBCs): > 2 = trauma to kidneys, renal diseases, excess aspirin, infection, menstrual contamination • WBCs: > 4 UTI, fever, strenuous exercise, lupus, nephritis, renal disease • Casts: Fever, renal diseases, heart failure
Ultrasound abdomen/pelvis	76700	$158	• Determines presence of masses
CT scan abdomen/pelvis	74178	$818	• Useful for diagnosing tumors, obstructions, cysts, hematomas, abscess, bleeding perforation, calculi, fibroids, and other pathologic conditions that appear in the abdomen and pelvis.

CLINICAL DECISION MAKING

Case Study Analysis

The advanced practice nurse (APN) discusses the possibility of pregnancy after the examination and the patient beings to cry and admits to having a boyfriend with whom she has had intercourse. The patient agrees to have a urine pregnancy test and this is positive. There is no abdominal pain to suggest an ectopic pregnancy or an infection. Other etiologies of vomiting are eliminated in the history and examination. The patient agrees to discuss the pregnancy with her mother with the APN present. They are referred to a local obstetrics and gynecology clinic for further evaluation.

Diagnosis: *Pregnancy*

FURTHER READING

Bickley, L. S., & Szilagyi, P. G. (2009). *Bates' guide to physical examination and history taking.* Philadelphia, PA: Wolters Kluwer Lippincott Williams & Wilkins.

Dains, J., Bauman, L., & Scheibel, P. (2007). *Advanced health assessment and clinical diagnosis in primary care.* St. Louis, MO: Elseiver Mosby.

Goolsby, M. J. (2011). *Advanced assessment interpreting findings and formulating differential diagnoses.* Philadelphia, PA: F.A. Davis Company.

Kee, J. L. (2005). *Handbook of laboratory & diagnostic tests* (5th ed.). Upper Sadle River, NJ: Prentice Hall.

WRIST PAIN

Case Presentation: *A 43-year-old woman presents to your clinic with a complaint of wrist pain for 2 days.*

INTRODUCTION TO COMPLAINT

Wrist pain may be caused by trauma; overuse through activities, such as knitting or typing; inflammatory disorders, such as arthritis; or neurological problems, such as nerve entrapment.

Acute Pain

Duration of pain observed is less than 2 weeks.

- Trauma
- Inflammation from gout, osteoarthritis, or rheumatoid arthritis

Subacute and Chronic Pain

Duration of pain observed is 2 weeks to 3 months (subacute) or more than 3 months (chronic).

- Prior acute trauma
- Chronic repetitive trauma or overuse
- Degenerative disease, such as osteoarthritis
- Connective tissue disorders, such as rheumatoid arthritis

HISTORY OF COMPLAINT

Symptomatology

Ask about the following characteristics of each symptom using open-ended questions:

- Onset: sudden or gradual
- Trauma: If yes, have the patient describe specifics of fall or other injury
- Location
- Timing: Is the pain greater at a specific time of the day?
- Severity on a scale of 0 to 10
- Quality: Is the pain burning, aching, stabbing, hot, cold?
- Continual or intermittent pain
- Weakness during specific movements
- Instability: Does the wrist "give out"?
- Sensation: Numbness, tingling

- Stiffness
- Functional disability: Does the pain interfere with usual activities?
- Skin color or temperature changes
- Recent trauma
- Course: worsening, improving, or stable?
- Exacerbating factors
- Alleviating factors
- Self-treatment: What has been tried? What was the result?
- Occupational and recreational activities
- Recent unusual activities like overtime, repainting the house
- Dominant hand: If patient endorses ambidexterity, ask which hand is used to write.
- Previous occurrences of similar complaint

Directed Questions to Ask

- Can you describe the injury from the beginning?
- Was there immediate pain?
- Was there immediate swelling?
- How has your pain changed since the injury?
- Can you point to the area of pain?
- Do you have weakness of your hand grip?
- Does the wrist or hand just give way?
- Do you have any numbness or tingling of the hand or wrist?
- If this is present, can you show me where it is?
- Does the wrist or hand feel cold?
- Have you had to change your normal activities?
- Do you do any type of work or hobby with your hands?
- Does your family have any history of arthritis or joint disease?

Assessment: Cardinal Signs and Symptoms

- Etiology
- Injury with swelling
- Sprain/fracture
- No trauma, heat, or swelling
- Gout
- Arthritis
- Numbness and tingling
- Nerve injury, carpal tunnel
- Weakness

Medical History: General

- Medications, including supplements and over-the-counter (OTC) medications
- Rheumatologic, inflammatory, or neuromuscular conditions
- Past trauma
- Any family history of rheumatologic, inflammatory, or neuromuscular conditions

Medical History: Specific to Complaint

- Any previous history of joint pain
- Any family history of gout, arthritis, or inflammatory joint diseases such as rheumatoid arthritis

PHYSICAL EXAMINATION
Vital Signs

- Blood pressure
- Heart rate
- Respiratory rate
- Weight
- Level of pain

General Appearance

- Comfort
- Nutritional status
- Hygiene level
- Hydration

Hand and Wrist Exam

Inspection

Observe the patient's upper extremities bilaterally from fingertip to elbow and note:

- Skin color and turgor
- Presence or absence of normal hair growth
- Swelling or nodules
- Skin tightness or looseness
- Deformity
- Symmetry: dominant side is usually larger and stronger
- Ulnar or radial deviation
- Position
- Contractures
- Ease, smoothness, and dexterity of movement

Palpation

- Observe the patient's face for signs of discomfort during palpation rather than observing the area palpated
- Palpate hand, wrist, and forearm
- Palpate corresponding areas on contralateral extremity to note any differences
- Note temperature of skin
- Note any "bogginess" of tissue, especially tendons or ligaments
- Note any discrete firm masses: are they moveable or fixed?
- Crepitus?
- Joint laxity?
- Swelling: discrete or diffuse?

Wrist Specific

Scaphoid: Use thumb on "anatomic snuffbox" and index finger on thenar eminence. Tenderness may indicate scaphoid injury.

Passive Range of Motion

Move the patient through range of motion, and watch patient's face for any sign of discomfort.

- Spasticity: difficulty in moving joint
- Crepitus
- Snapping or popping? A brief snap or pop that is only momentarily uncomfortable is not a concern.

Movement
Observe the patient during active range of motion.

- FINGER: flexion, extension
- WRIST: flexion, extension, ulnar deviation, radial deviation, pronation with flexed elbow, supination with flexed elbow
- ELBOW: flexion, extension, pronation, supination

Observe functional ability as the patient performs.

- Fine pinch: picking up a paper clip
- Flat pinch: holding a key to unlock a door
- Tripod grip: using a pen
- Wide grip: grasping the circumference of a mug
- Power grip: holding a hammer

Tinel's test: Light tapping over volar wrist; sensation of tingling, electrical pain or "pins and needles" may indicate nerve compression as in carpal tunnel syndrome.

Phalen's test: Have patient flex wrists and hold for 60 seconds. Sensations of tingling or numbness may indicate nerve compression. Negative results do not rule out nerve compression.

Ulnar Side
- Tendinopathy, subluxation, fibrocartilagenous injuries, especially from repetitive actions (from racquet sports, excessive computer keyboard/mouse use)
- Triangular fibrocartilage complex injury; suspect this if your dominant finding is ulnar-side wrist pain, or find instability of wrist. Most commonly occurs from trauma. May be caused by overuse injury in occupations like carpentry.

Radial Side
- Scaphoid fracture; frequent after moderate trauma; tenderness at anatomic snuffbox. May cause avascular necrosis later. X-rays are usually initially negative.
- deQuervain's tenosynovitis. Pain with grasp or pinch. Usually caused by overuse.
- Osteoarthritis is rarely seen in the wrist unless there is a history of previous injury. If there is osteoarthritis of the wrist, you will see prominent carpometacarpal and metacarpophalangeal joint pain.
- Rheumatoid arthritis frequently affects the wrist, is symmetrical and bilateral, and presents with ulnar deviation of fingers and metacarpals.
- Inflammatory conditions, such as infections or gout, are rare in the wrist. If suspected, examine and aspirate.

Volar Side
- Carpal or ulnar neuropathy: symptoms are worse at night; pain at hypothenar eminence (if ulnar). Positive Tinel's or Phalen's signs; wasting of thenar or hypothenar eminence
- Hamate bone fracture can mimic pain from strain/sprain. Pain is usually observed over the hypothenar eminence.

Dorsal Side
- Ganglion cyst: discrete, spheroid mass, somewhat movable, not hard nor fixed; often returns after aspiration; may require referral to hand surgeon
- Degenerative osteophyte formation, usually occurs at base of second and third metacarpals; "carpal boss": fixed, bony mass

- Kienbock's disease of lunate: slow onset; chronic; mild swelling; progressive dorsal wrist pain
- Forearm tendinopathy or "intersection syndrome" is caused by friction where portions of the abductor pollicis longus and extensor pollicis brevis pass over the extensor carpi radialis longus and extensor carpi radialis brevis. Pain over distal, dorsal forearm, especially with wrist extension. Etiology is most often from overuse. Crepitation or tendonous "creaking" (use stethoscope) may be heard over area.

CASE STUDY
History

Question	Response
How did the pain begin?	*Suddenly*
How did the injury happen?	*I was walking my lively young dog on a leash when the dog suddenly leapt to chase a squirrel. During the dog's maneuvers I tripped over the leash, fell, and attempted to break my fall with outstretched right hand, and I landed on hard-packed dirt.*
Where is the pain?	*Right side of wrist/base of palm*
Is the pain greater at a specific time of the day?	*No*
On a scale of 0 to 10, 10 being the most severe, how much pain do you have?	*4 to 6*
Is the pain burning, aching, stabbing, hot, cold?	*Aching*
Continual or intermittent pain?	*Continual*
Weakness during specific movements?	*No loss of strength, but painful*
Does the wrist "give out"?	*No*
Do you have any numbness or tingling?	*No*
Do you have any stiffness?	*No*
Does the pain interfere with usual activities?	*I avoid any activity that increase the pain, especially gripping objects*
Have you had any skin color or temperature changes?	*No*
Has the pain worsened, improved, or is it stable?	*Stable*
What makes it worse?	*Using my wrist*
What makes it feel better; what have you tried?	*Acetaminophen or ibuprofen at OTC doses is moderately helpful*

Question	*Response*
What are your occupational and recreational activities?	*I am an interior designer and use my computer and mouse extensively, which has been painful since the injury. And I like gardening, which I have not been able to do since the injury.*
Any recent unusual activities like overtime, repainting the house?	*No*
Which is your dominant hand?	*Right*
Any previous occurrences of similar complaint?	*No*

Physical Examination Findings

Observe a diffuse ecchymosis over proximal thenar eminence on the right hand. The patient moves her right hand and wrist gingerly. The right wrist appears mildly swollen during extension. She complains of increased pain when gripping with right hand, and with firm palpation of thenar eminence. She is mildly tender in the anatomical snuffbox. Otherwise there are no remarkable findings on the right side, and her left is normal.

DIFFERENTIAL DIAGNOSES

Differential Diagnosis	Trauma	Osteoarthritis	Rheumatoid Arthritis	Gout	Ganglion Cyst	Nerve Compression	Repetitive Trauma/Overuse
Onset	Sudden	Rarely	Possibly	Possibly	No	Rarely	No
Bilateral	Variable	Rarely	Yes	No	No	Unlikely	Possibly dominant side most affected
Deformity	Variable	Hypertrophy of thumb, distal interphalangeal, metacarpo-phalangeal, carpometacarpal joints	Hypertrophy of proximal inter-phalangeal joints; ulnar deviation	Swelling	Swelling	No	Rarely; muscle wasting if chronic
Warmth	Variable	Unlikely	Yes	Yes	No	No	No
Stiffness	Variable	Yes	Yes	No	No	No	No

DIAGNOSTIC EXAMINATION

Examination	Procedure Code	Cost	Indication/Interpretation
X-ray, plain film	733120	$200	<ul><li>Inexpensive</li><li>Fairly low radiation exposure</li><li>Correct positioning is essential for accurate diagnosis</li><li>Initial evaluation: posteroanterior, lateral, and oblique; if concern for scaphoid fracture, add scaphoid view</li></ul>Trauma, weakness, locking; may reveal calcification or fracture
MRI	74200	$850	<ul><li>Expensive</li><li>No exposure to radiation</li><li>Best for soft tissue assessment (ganglia, tendinitis, effusions)</li></ul>
CT	74202	$750 to $950	<ul><li>Expensive</li><li>Exposes patient to increased radiation, although lower radiation techniques are increasingly used</li><li>Useful for assessment of bone healing</li></ul>

CLINICAL DECISION MAKING

Case Study

The patient has a 2-day history of acute trauma, and her examination shows predominantly radial-sided symptoms. Although tenderness at the anatomic snuffbox is mild, you are concerned as you know the scaphoid bone is a common area for fracture after a fall with outstretched hand. Accordingly, you order plain films for your patient, including posterior–anterior, lateral, oblique, and scaphoid views. The imaging returns negative. You know that the negative x-rays do not rule out an occult or hairline fracture, especially of the scaphoid bone. Future imaging will be necessary before final diagnosis.

Diagnosis: Wrist pain, possibly contusion. Tenderness of the scaphoid area with negative x-ray does not rule out a fracture. Consider referral to a hand specialist. Another alternative is to repeat the x-ray in 2 weeks to see whether an occult fracture is identified.

INDEX